"If you are bruised and broken, Kobe's bo[...] of this book, you will learn how to transfo[...] umph, your pain into purpose, and your scars will become a testimony of God's grace. Healing awaits you."

—DR. DERWIN GRAY, LEAD PASTOR AND COFOUNDER OF TRANSFORMATION CHURCH

"This book is absolutely incredible. Kobe Campbell marries trauma principles and theological insight to help readers answer one of the most painful questions a person can ever ask. *Why Am I Like This?* is a must-read for anyone looking for evidence-based resources rooted in tenderness and grace."

—DANIEL G. AMEN, MD, FOUNDER OF AMEN CLINICS AND AUTHOR OF *CHANGE YOUR BRAIN EVERY DAY*

"From the first page, I literally couldn't stop reading. This is one of the best therapy books I've read and definitely the best Christian therapy book. I found myself cringing because I could see and feel so much of my own story as Kobe shared hers. It was so vulnerable and relatable. This book is an answered prayer for people longing to understand how God responds to their mental and emotional health. A must-read!"

—TANA AMEN, BSN AND RN, VICE PRESIDENT OF AMEN CLINICS AND AUTHOR OF *THE RELENTLESS COURAGE OF A SCARED CHILD*

"Kobe wrote the book I've been praying to be on the shelves of bookstores for years. She has an impeccable gift with the way she puts words together. Every sentence is approachable yet hard-hitting. This book is validating, educational, and talking about the underlying pain many of us have experienced and are experiencing. This is the content I believe so many people, especially Christians, have been seeking. She is giving those of us who have been silenced by, and in, the church a language to express our experiences. Let this book cover you and comfort you in the way you have been longing for!"

—CHRISTINA WILCOX, AUTHOR OF *TAKE CARE OF YOUR TYPE*

"Kobe Campbell gives us permission to ask the question underneath the question of Why Am I Like This?: What happened to me? With skill and compassion, Campbell disarms the shame that chains our stories, offering us rest and lasting relief instead. You'll see yourself in these pages, and you'll also glimpse the kind eyes of God looking back at you with love."

—K.J. RAMSEY, THERAPIST AND AUTHOR OF *THE BOOK OF COMMON COURAGE* AND *THE LORD IS MY COURAGE*

WHY AM I LIKE THIS?

WHY AM I LIKE THIS?

HOW TO BREAK CYCLES, HEAL FROM TRAUMA, AND RESTORE YOUR FAITH

KOBE CAMPBELL

MACC, LCMHC

W PUBLISHING GROUP

AN IMPRINT OF THOMAS NELSON

Why Am I Like This?

Published in Nashville, Tennessee, by W Publishing, an imprint of Thomas Nelson.

Published in association with The Bindery Agency, www.TheBinderyAgency.com.

Thomas Nelson titles may be purchased in bulk for educational, business, fundraising, or sales promotional use. For information, please email SpecialMarkets@ThomasNelson.com.

Any internet addresses, phone numbers, or company or product information printed in this book are offered as a resource and are not intended in any way to be or to imply an endorsement by Thomas Nelson, nor does Thomas Nelson vouch for the existence, content, or services of these sites, phone numbers, companies, or products beyond the life of this book.

Some personal names and identifying details have been changed to protect the privacy of the individuals involved.

The information in this book has been carefully researched by the author and is intended to be a source of information only. While the methods contained herein can and do work, readers are urged to consult with their physicians or other professional advisors to address any medical issues. The author and the publisher assume no responsibility for any injuries suffered or damages or losses incurred during or as a result of the use or application of the information contained herein.

ISBN 978-0-7852-9644-7 (audiobook)
ISBN 978-0-7852-9643-0 (eBook)
ISBN 978-0-7852-9642-3 (softcover)

Library of Congress Control Number: 2022945068

Printed in the United States of America

23 24 25 26 27 LBC 6 5 4 3 2

*To my incredible husband, Kyle, I couldn't
have done this without you.
To my brave clients, thank you for letting me
experience the miracle of your stories.
To every version of myself I struggled to love, your
courage turned all that pain into something beautiful.*

CONTENTS

CONTENTS

WILL I EVER FEEL FREE?

I fumbled over my keys as my fingers finally found the right one for my front door. The world was swaying, but that was no surprise to me; that's what happens when you've had six shots and snorted a couple of Percocet. I wasn't entirely sure how I got home, but I remembered feeling relatively safe during the drive. The door clicked open with the turn of my wrist, and I gracelessly tripped into the common area, then walked into my room. I touched my lips to test how drunk I was. They were numb.

I chuckled. "Yep, you're *drunk* drunk, Kobe." I plopped onto my bed fully clothed.

As my body sank into the mattress, my heart went with it. The room was silent, and I knew with silence comes pain. Before I could turn on my TV for background noise or blast some music to distract my mind, the memories started. Every heartbreak, betrayal, dissolved friendship, and criticism surfaced from the back of my mind and sprinted their way to the front of my consciousness: the time my boyfriend cheated on me, the jokes about my being the "bad twin," the friends I'd introduced to one another who no longer wanted to be friends with me. Every moment swirled in the room. Even worse were the moments where I was the one to break my own heart. Thoughts about going further than I wanted to with a guy I barely liked started to play in my mind. My stomach twisted as I remembered the shame of seeing him out in public. He never texted me back but told all his friends about it. I was so ashamed. I just wanted to be loved.

Why doesn't anyone want to love me? I asked myself in the silence of my heart. *Why does everyone leave me?* These questions unveiled a pain no drink could numb and no drug could hide—pain deep in my bones.

With an energetic determination, I decided I didn't want to live anymore. After twenty years of living, the bullying, insecurities, racism, sexism, heartbreak, and crippling loneliness I'd experienced felt unending. Life was a cycle of trying to get people to love me only to find out they wouldn't. I was done. Life was more bad than good. It wasn't worth living.

At the time I believed in something spiritual—I just wasn't sure what. Growing up, I'd gone to church every Sunday, and I felt the burn of longing in my heart during the altar call, when the pastor talked about being free and starting a new life. I even built up the courage to make my way to the front of the church a few times, to "give my life to Christ." I accepted Jesus into my heart—and then life went back to normal.

I thought about those memories as I lay in my room. I felt embarrassed. Silly for thinking that whoever was running this show cared about me. No one loved me. *Not even me.*

As I snapped back to the present, my eyes wandered to a bottle of vodka I'd left on my desk before I went out, then darted to the orange bottle of Percocet the dentist had given me a week before my wisdom tooth extraction. My appointment got canceled after I'd already filled the prescription. I should never have had them.

I took a deep breath, then grabbed my pills and tossed four or five of them into my mouth as I threw my head back. The plan was to take them in one smooth swallow, but instead I ended up half chewing them because they were so big. I picked up the vodka and chugged it until my lips burned from the alcohol.

"If I'm going out, I am *not* going out in pain," I said to myself, laughing. I'd been laughed at my whole life—why not join in?

I immediately felt tired and a little nauseous. There had been so many nights when I'd thought to myself, *You know, it wouldn't be so bad if I didn't wake up tomorrow morning.* This time it wouldn't just be a flippant expression of hopelessness. I grabbed a piece of paper to write a letter to my twin sister, to tell her I was sorry for leaving her. I knew she'd be devastated. I also wrote a small note apologizing to my roommates and nestled my head into my pillow as I snuggled under my blanket. This was it. I felt myself drifting into what I thought would be a never-ending sleep.

Then my phone chimed.

I jumped up, startled by the sound in the silence. I looked at my phone, and it said I had a message from Brent (my friend who led a Bible study on campus). I opened the text, and my heart stopped.

"I was praying, and the Lord told me that you took some pills and drank some vodka. He told me to tell you to rip up the letter you wrote because you're not going to die. He has a purpose for your life, and you shouldn't go to sleep."

I was beyond shocked; I was terrified, embarrassed, and confused. My eyes ran over each letter of each word again and again. I couldn't understand it. This wasn't possible. Still, in the chaos of confusion, I felt one thing I hadn't felt in so long: hope. I had this unexplainable desire to smile in the midst of utter shock and denial as I attempted to end my life.

Someone *saw* me.

Still, hope wasn't something I was used to holding on to, so I tried to shrug off the absolutely miraculous moment by telling myself I was just high and hallucinating. I didn't respond. Instead, I turned my phone off, turned over, and went to sleep. It's amazing how, when sadness accumulates, it hardens the heart to God's goodness and mercy.

Yet, He persists.

A loud *ding* sliced through the silence of my room.

My body froze. *I know I just turned my phone off. What the heck?* I flipped my pillow over and, sure enough, my phone was on, screen bright as can be, with a notification that said, "Message from Brent."

"God said stay up," it read. I couldn't believe it.

Over the next hour, Brent told me about how God loved me and how He had a magnificent plan for my life. I read one part of Brent's message over and over again: "longs to be with you." I'd seen those words arranged exactly as I read them, but they had always been hidden in stanzas of poetry or written in fiction fantasies—they were never for me. No one had ever longed to be with *me*.

I vacillated between letting my heart be carried away by the hope that there was a God who loved and saw me, and being embarrassed and ashamed that someone knew I wanted to die. Between two and seven o'clock that morning, I tried to turn my phone off several times. It just wouldn't stay off. I can't explain it. Or maybe I can; I knew it was God. Brent texted me the entire time, relentlessly sharing Bible verses and encouragement, insisting that I come with him to church in the morning.

By the time day broke, I had grown tired of resisting God's love—a weariness I'll always welcome. I built up the courage to go to church with Brent after years of only going when my parents made me. When we walked in, I felt something I'd never experienced before. It was the burning I felt in my heart as a child during altar calls, but instead of a flame, it was a furnace. I heard a voice in my heart say that I was loved and that He was waiting for me. I knew it was God. I knew it was my Daddy; He hadn't forgotten me. My knees buckled, and I lay on the ground the entire service. The Lord's love covered me like a weighted blanket.

That day I said yes to doing life with Christ.

In that moment, every single depressive symptom and anxious thought disappeared. Every shameful moment evaporated, and every memory of heartbreak disintegrated. I felt free and unburdened.

For about a week.

In the months and years that followed, I struggled to hold on to the gospel. If God conquered sin and brokenness on the cross, why was I still dealing with painful memories? If my cares were cast on Him, why was I still anxious? I truly loved God but still felt crippling shame.

Why am I like this? I wondered. *Why can't I shake the pain of my past?* I thought the hope of the gospel was freedom and the fruit of its presence in my life was joy. But here I was, too anxious to call on Jesus and trapped in cycles of despair.

We All Need Healing

Though I wake in fear
I sleep in peace
Cause when I pray

You meet my needs
When I cry
You whisper back
When I kneel
You hold my hand
In my weakness
You are my strength
When I'm stubborn
You give tenderness
When I run
You're always near
In my distress you catch every tear

I wrote this poem as a prophetic hope. I was neck-deep in a depressive episode. My head knew the truth of God's love for me, but my heart had forgotten its touch. Even if you haven't lived under the weight of depression, you've likely experienced this reality. After praying, reading my Bible, and doing all the "right things," I was still stuck in cycles of sadness, self-loathing, self-betrayal, and self-sabotage. Something just wasn't clicking. I knew there was more to life, and I wanted to experience it, but there seemed to be this invisible barrier that kept me from consistently living it out.

I would change for a few months or weeks at a time. But then I'd find my way back to the old patterns that made the truth of God's love feel like a dream I was chasing rather than a reality I lived in. I couldn't see that the pain of my past was keeping me from living in the freedom God had for me. I didn't realize that the fragmented memories of moments I wanted to forget were clues to why I felt so stuck. Though I said yes to a new life in Christ, I still needed Him to hold my hand through deep emotional, psychological, and spiritual healing.

Maybe you're like me and you've grown tired of living in cycles you want to break, or you want the abundant life in Christ that you know you were created for. Maybe you want to understand why you are the way you are and rest in the fact that you're accepted by God fully. Maybe you're not sure what you want; you just know that you need healing and have no idea how to embark on the journey. I know how you feel.

In my personal journey with mental health and in my professional practice of providing trauma therapy, I've encountered an overwhelming truth. Many of us have been taught by the church and the world at large, both explicitly and implicitly, that the mental and emotional pain that come from trauma are character problems and moral failings. They are seen as personal flaws marked by laziness, ignorance, immaturity, and a lack of gratitude. We're taught that we can outrun, outlearn, and outearn the anguish. We begin to believe that more status, knowledge, and resources will give us the key to unlocking a life where we are immune to our own emotional reality.

But such a life doesn't exist. We know that because of the life of Jesus.

In Jesus' relationships and ministry, He utilized a full range of emotions to live a perfect, blameless, and holy life—a full range of emotions many of us have turned our backs on. But we'll need these emotions to live in intimate unity with God and others.

We've been taught that if we get too close to our emotions, we'll be consumed by them and miss our healing. I'm here to tell you that if you don't get close *enough*, you surely will.

The small things that bother us point to the big wounds that cripple us. I think the greatest barrier to healing is embarrassment. Many of us are too afraid to share the truth about the big and little things that truly wound us. We're afraid to share about the facial expression someone made that caused us to feel shame about sharing our honest thoughts. We're scared to speak of the person who touched us inappropriately, because we anticipate blame. In all of this, the terror lives on, isolating us and baiting us into a narrative of hopelessness, while whispering lies of God's disappointment and anger toward us.

A LITTLE ABOUT ME

After my miraculous moment with God, I just wanted to move on. I wanted to stop talking about the past. I wanted to hurry up and live a new life. But God kept bringing me back to moments I wanted to forget. He kept drawing my mind and heart to remember the moments that made me feel shameful and worthless. For so long I thought it was punishment, because it felt like torture. Little did I know, it was God walking me through the process of healing.

In my therapist's office, I came to know the deepest love and acceptance I'd ever experienced. It gave me a tangible reference for the attentive, gentle wisdom of the Holy Spirit. Through my therapist, my view of God as my advocate blossomed. After years of receiving therapy, my heart ached to be a part of how God showed His love, mercy, and tenderness in the mental health field. So, after getting my bachelor's in psychology, I attended Gordon-Conwell Theological Seminary to get my degree in Christian counseling as a licensed clinical mental health counselor (LCMHC). I have since developed a specialty in trauma through modalities like EMDR (Eye Movement Desensitization and Reprocessing), Psychodrama, and Somatic Experiencing. It was and still is important to me to marry the perspectives of therapy and theology, knowing that both disciplines reflect the love of God. If we want to love, serve, and honor our neighbors and ourselves, we have to understand the beautifully intricate way that God has made us. My practice, The Healing Circle Therapy & Wellness Center, specializes in just that—helping people heal from their traumas and access abounding love for themselves and others as they journey through the wilderness of their pain.

OUR JOURNEY TOGETHER

In these pages, you'll find that the patterns that you can't shake aren't character flaws. The low self-esteem you can't break free from isn't moral failure. The depression that keeps coming back isn't a lack of faith, or laziness. The relationships that keep ending with abandonment aren't God punishing you. They're evidence of trauma—deep wounds longing to be healed and crying out for the divine touch of God Himself.

We'll begin our journey by getting a clear understanding of what trauma is. Then we'll uncover how our negative patterns affect us, explore how our past affects our present, discover how fear limits us, and clarify the identity-wounds that trauma creates. After we gain a clear understanding of how our wounds affect us, we'll dive into what to do with that knowledge as we take courageous steps toward the intimacy, presence, and belonging we were designed to experience. We'll pick up some heavy weights, but we'll also learn how to lay them down, as we take hold of lighthearted laughter and experience the freedom our hearts have been longing for.

Throughout the book I'll be sharing real stories. Some will be my own, and others will be of clients, whom I've renamed for the sake of confidentiality. I decided to give each person an African name. As a first-generation Ghanaian American, I rarely heard stories of heartbreak, hope, or redemption attached to a name that sounded like mine or anyone in my family. Our names were too complicated, too thick on the tongue to a world that rarely stops to listen to the nuance of our stories. The capacity to heal is ours, too, and I'm excited to share a small part of my culture with you.

This book is a literary representation of my journey of healing and restoration. My path included deep Scripture study, psychoeducation, and expressions of the cocktail of emotions and experiences I sometimes brought to the Father and other times hid from Him. You'll read my clinical thoughts, my theological findings, and my personal poetry. This isn't just a journey of education; it's also one of community. Healing is not a static destination, and I'm not ashamed to admit that some days I still wrestle with the ghosts of my past. On those days, I'm comforted by how loudly the hard-fought truths I've discovered in therapy and Scripture drown out the lies. My prayer is that this will become your experience too.

My story of coming to know God is not unique. It's miraculous, but that same miraculous power is accessible to you. Right now. Right here. This moment is God sending you a message, relentlessly reaching out to you like Brent did to me. Though you may not feel it, God is meeting your despair with gentleness and incredible hope.

Healing won't look like what you thought it would, but it will come, and it will be beautiful.

part one

UNDERSTANDING OUR PAIN

chapter one

TRAUMA: HOW DID MY PAST AFFECT ME?

I took a seat after grabbing some pizza from the cafeteria line. I could tell I'd just joined a serious conversation being had by the people already seated. I listened to them share about their painful childhood experiences. I was moved by their vulnerability and relieved to be surrounded by people who weren't afraid to talk about things I normally attached shame to. I sipped my lemonade as I contemplated whether I would jump in. I decided I would.

"I'm so sorry you went through that," I told a girl who just admitted that she'd struggled with suicidal thoughts in the past. "I know how that feels. I remember when, after my high school boyfriend broke up with me, I felt so rejected and heartbroken. It was the first time I wondered if I deserved to live."

The table grew silent. I paused to take a sip of my drink before I continued to share—but I didn't get that chance. Before I could start my next statement, a girl to the right of me blurted out, "That's it?

You really need to grow thicker skin. Focus on what God has for you *now*. You're not in high school anymore. Don't you know Scripture tells us to forget the past and focus on what is ahead?"

My skin grew hot, and my heart shriveled as she spoke. I was deflated. Once again, Scripture was being used to invalidate my experiences. Validation was reserved only for people whose pain was worthy, and mine wasn't. How was I supposed to find refuge in something that was always used as a weapon against me in my weakest moments?

At the time, I would have said I was hurt, maybe even ashamed. But now, with almost a decade of therapy under my belt and a full view of how that tiny seed of dismissal grew into a mighty oak of shame, I can say with full confidence I was traumatized by that moment and others like it. Even as a trauma therapist, it feels incredibly scary and vulnerable to say that such a common, everyday moment traumatized me. The Enemy purposefully ties our deepest pain to the most normal and mundane moments of our lives, forcing us to endure ridicule if we dare to tell the truth. How easy it is to lie about what hurt us when we know the truth will offer up a double serving of shame.

I know I'm guilty of exaggerating moments of betrayal and hurt for fear that the person on the listening end won't find the same significance in the seemingly small moments I found devastating. I also know I'm not alone. Healing is complicated and messy. And honestly, it sucks until it doesn't.

The word *trauma* in Greek simply translates to the word "wound."[1] Nowadays when we hear the word *trauma* we think of sexual abuse, domestic violence, soldiers at war, natural disasters, and death—all of which *are* trauma but don't fully encompass the vast experiences that also fit under its definition. Trauma is also bullying, being embarrassed by a partner, betrayal from a friend, physical or emotional abandonment by a parent, financial insecurity, religious fearmongering, verbal abuse, rejection from your kids, psychological abuse, loneliness in marriage, a difficult birthing experience, being dismissed at work, and so much more. Trauma is any moment or series of moments that have lasting negative effects on our physical, emotional, spiritual, mental, relational, financial, and/or social well-being.

Although both bullying and sexual abuse are examples of trauma, we often try to put one above the other—but we can't and shouldn't. They both wound deeply. They both shape our identity. They distort our perception of ourselves, our reality, and the God who created us.

Before my suicide attempt, my trauma was from being bullied for having dark skin, being constantly compared to my twin sister, losing close friendships, being sexually assaulted, and the loneliness that came from trying to keep it all a secret as a teenager and young adult. My trauma created patterns of hiding, suppressing my feelings, and only engaging with people when I was in a good mood or accomplished something. I was in a cycle I wanted to escape.

This is a reality I see in many of the clients I serve. A reality that leads to questions like:

"How do I stop retreating?"

"How do I share my feelings?"

"How do I express my pain and feel okay when people see me upset?"

The answer to all these is: you address your trauma.

Trauma is any moment or series of moments that have lasting negative effects on our physical, emotional, spiritual, mental, relational, financial, and/or social well-being.

IT *WAS* THAT BAD

When I tell my clients that the experiences they've had are traumatic, the first thing I encounter is denial.

"No, no, it wasn't that bad!" or "I don't think it was trauma. That sounds too intense."

My response is usually, "It is. That's why you're here."

Even when we resist the idea that the intangible and interpersonal things we've suffered through are trauma, deep down we know it's true. Without language to name it, we feel it in our hearts, sense it in our bodies, and see it in the inescapable patterns and cycles we engage in daily. Because we are often too scared to investigate the unshakable thoughts, inescapable sensations, and unbreakable patterns, we turn our backs on the pain of our past experiences and run as fast as we can away from it—only to run right back into it through the patterns that protect us for a moment but estrange us from love and peace for years. It's hard to let go of the patterns that are both self-protective and self-destructive. It's easy to run from our problems when the world rewards the busyness that distracts us from seeing the true state of our heart. We know deep down that the accolades only highlight the anger and disappointment we feel toward ourselves when we *don't* achieve something. We know it because guilt washes over us even in moments of celebration. Though life appears "good" and nothing looks "wrong," a looming sense of loneliness and sadness blankets our days. We know we can't outrun the pain, but we still try to.

Some of us have no clue what is at the root of our negative thoughts, feelings, and actions. Others of us know exactly what lies beneath the surface, because we're haunted by memories and fragments of memories we don't want to talk about or acknowledge.

We're stuck between the option of confessing that the things the world calls "small" have big impacts on us or suffering in silence with a smile on our face. Many of us choose the latter. It often feels like the world, the church, and even God would *prefer* the latter from us.

You know in the corners of your heart there are moments that need to be seen even if you don't want to look at them. It's true for all of us. It can feel incredibly shameful to say we believe in Jesus and yet are so wounded. Christians are supposed to have unwavering hope, right?

When I experienced my first depressive episode as a new and eager Christian, I thought it was safe to share what I was going through. However, I was told by a leader that my depression was ruining my witness. "Who would want to follow a Jesus who has depressed followers?" this leader said. I still tear up thinking about that moment—and all the moments of lonely, pain-filled silence that followed it. I vowed to never let anyone see me sad again.

If they were disappointed in me, how much more was God?

That's trauma.

LOOKING AT OUR PAIN

Many of us spend our lives distracting ourselves from our pain by serving and giving to others, all the while hoping our altruism will scrub the stains of sadness from our soul. The fear that motivates us robs us of the deep joy of service and connection, while helping us maintain an image of humility and assurance.

Our trauma has a way of terrorizing us, keeping us in fear while baiting us with the lie that we will never experience freedom. In our fear and denial, we wonder:

Was that thing that happened to me really that bad?
What can God do about it?
That was so long ago, why can't I get over it?
Maybe life isn't that bad. I'm overreacting.
Maybe I don't need to talk about this.

In our hopelessness and terror, we ask ourselves:

Will this pain last forever?
Will anyone ever love me?
Why does everyone leave me?
Why does my faith feel useless when I need it most?
Is God disappointed in me?

Silent questions like these can ring so loudly that it's almost impossible to hear the gentle voice of the Father. Let's begin to unpack why.

WHAT IS TRAUMA?

What is trauma, really?

Trauma is the physical, emotional, and psychological response to a distressing event or experience. It's a deep wound from past events that affects how we perceive and experience the present and anticipate the future.

As a therapist, a question I often get is, "What's the difference between something that hurt you in the moment and something that is traumatic?" We can distinguish between trauma and a painful moment based on how we respond to it and how it affects us in the future.

Painful moments affect us, but they don't leave us with intense fear and a sense of helplessness that extends significantly past the moment of pain. They don't negatively shape how we view our identity, perceive others, and anticipate the future. If an experience does, then it's trauma. Trauma primes our mind, body, and spirit for perpetual fear, trapping us physically, emotionally, spiritually, and relationally in loops of pain, even when that moment is long gone.

Trauma is the sexual assault you never told anyone about, *and* it's your friend making mean comments under the guise of a joke. It's years of your spouse pulling out bank statements to make you account for every cent you spent, *and* it's being in a horrific car accident. Trauma is middle school bullying *and* domestic abuse. It's growing up in foster care, *and* it's being beat relentlessly for small mistakes. It's hearing your mother call your sister beautiful every day, while your heart felt the silence of her compliments toward you. It's being emotionally abandoned when you trusted someone with your heart. It's your parents telling you that you were stupid and useless. Trauma is having a friend walk away when you needed them. It's growing up with financial insecurity, *and* it's growing up with all the money in the world but no one to spend time with you. All trauma is deeply personal and, in many ways, is undefinable apart from the complexities of an individual and their personal values.

Our society often likes to classify things as "big T" traumas or "little t" traumas, to demonstrate which trauma is worse.[2] The truth is trauma is trauma, whether it's obvious to the eye or not. The only value in distinguishing the types of trauma is in helping people see the many ways it can manifest in our lives. The part of your brain that processes physical pain is the same part that processes emotional and relational pain. Abandonment activates the same networks in the brain as a punch in the face would. Pain is pain to the body and the brain; the only question is how aware of that reality we allow ourselves to be. It helps no one to rank traumas based on how big or little they are. Everyone comes in last place in the pain Olympics.

Clarifying this is so important because I've sat in my office and consoled clients who heard phrases like, "Get over it," "It wasn't that bad," and "You're being dramatic, so many people have it worse than you." Years of hearing these comments have made them afraid to be honest about their experiences, and without that safety to be honest and talk about it, there's little opportunity for healing.

My clients often share with me the secret promises they've made to themselves that come from being in unsafe spaces that have invalidated their pain: "I'll never let anyone see me sad or angry," or "I'll always put on a brave face." These promises offer the sense of safety they didn't feel with others but perpetuate the negative and destructive cycles that they sought out therapy to break in the first place.

Behind every promise to hide a vulnerable part of ourselves is almost always a traumatic moment that was invalidated.

It's amazing how comforting lies can be when we're in so much pain. We were made for deep and meaningful connection with others, God, and ourselves. I often remind my clients that there's a reason why isolation can be one of the highest forms of punishment. It shrinks the brain,[3] causing it to respond neurologically with a craving for connection the way our bodies hunger for food.[4] It starves us of our biological and emotional needs, while our souls wither away.

That, also, is trauma.

Different Types of Trauma

I remember one of my clients, Funmi (Foo-me), telling me that she had vowed to "never get attached to anyone." She decided that practicing non-attachment was best for her mental health. "If you don't get attached, they can't hurt you when they let you down," she argued.

Funmi struggled to see her trauma of emotional abandonment from her wealthy, still-married parents as valid, even though her vow to resist intimacy was a reflection of how deeply she had been wounded by them. She struggled to trust even the closest relationships in her life. When she went through a hard season of physical sickness, she needed support but couldn't bring herself to pick up the phone and call the people she knew would show up for her. Because of that insecurity, she once endured hours of lying on the floor when she'd fallen and even laid in a bed where she'd soiled herself after being unable to get to the bathroom.

Those were her wake-up calls. She lived with a motto of self-reliance and found it to be good and empowering. But when Funmi was in need, she discovered just how detrimental that pattern was. She couldn't understand how her relationship with her parents connected to her patterns of self-reliance and struggled even more to see her relationship with them as one that involved trauma.

"Some traumas look like big boulders," I told her. "They're clearly massive, they take up space, and they draw attention with a presence that's undeniable. Other traumas look like pebbles. Small rocks that are unassuming. In the moment, they cause pain, but in comparison to other things, they seem small and unimportant. Until one day you look up to find that all the pebbles you've collected over the years created the mass of a boulder." Though traumas can show up differently, it doesn't diminish the impact of them. But it does affect how we can detect them.

The "boulders" are what we would call *acute trauma*. They come from a single distressing event, like a fire that burned down our house, or violent physical abuse from a partner. The "pebbles" are what we call *chronic trauma*. They are repeated and prolonged, such as physical and emotional abuse in a home or relationship that's gone on for years. Acute traumas often shock and disorient us in the moment, while chronic traumas slowly chip away at our ability to hope, our confidence, and our sense of self.

Chronic trauma may look like a seemingly insignificant individual incident, but when you zoom out and look at the larger picture, a clear pattern appears. It often looks like parents not speaking well of you unless you won the game at school or made them proud with As on your report card. It's your family member constantly commenting on "how big you're getting" and your teacher calling you stupid in class. When those everyday wounds are inflicted, we begin to slowly shift into a fearful and anxious posture.

Trauma isn't limited to big boulders or small pebbles. Most of us have experienced a combination of the two. The combination of both acute and chronic trauma is what we call *complex trauma*. Each type and combination of trauma looks different and means different things for each person, but they all hurt our mind, body, and spirit the same.

Trauma Through the Lens of Scripture

Several years ago I felt the Lord prompt me to dive into Genesis for my personal Bible study. I began reading and noticed a deeper sense of attention emerge in my heart as I read Genesis 2 and 3. God was showing me something. I could feel it. I could see it.

When I had finished writing notes, I dropped my pen, scanned my chicken-scratch thoughts, and took a deep breath. *This is trauma*, I thought to myself.

The beginning of Genesis is where God sets the stage for His intention for creation. This includes humanity's relationship with nature, humanity's relationship with humanity, and humanity's relationship with God.

In this short passage we get a full picture of God's intention for humanity, for our lives. He created a world where we are near to Him, safe with Him, and loved by Him. A world where we are free, and He trusts us with His creation, to care for it. He created a world where we have freedom and can experience joy. He invites us into creativity and is deeply attuned to our needs. He provides for us in our loneliness, before we even notice that we are lonely. He designed us to be in relationship with others and celebrate our likeness and find beauty in our differences. He designed a world where we get to experience no shame toward ourselves and no shame toward others.[5]

This is the world we were meant to live in. A world that our hearts are still longing for. A world that many of us have seen so little of because in the next chapter, Genesis 3, trauma entered the story and shifted the narrative of creation.

I often ask people to begin reading Genesis 3 and identify where the trauma occurs in the narrative.

Now the serpent was more crafty than any of the wild animals the Lord God had made. He said to the woman, "Did God really say, 'You must not eat from any tree in the garden'?"

The woman said to the serpent, "We may eat fruit from the trees in the garden, but God did say, 'You must not eat fruit from the tree that is in the middle of the garden, and you must not touch it, or you will die.'"

"You will not certainly die," the serpent said to the woman. "For God knows that when you eat from it your eyes will be opened, and you will be like God, knowing good and evil."

When the woman saw that the fruit of the tree was good for food and pleasing to the eye, and also desirable for gaining wisdom, she took some and ate it. She also gave some to her husband, who was with her, and he ate it. Then the eyes of both of them were opened, and they realized they were naked; so they sewed fig leaves together and made coverings for themselves.

Then the man and his wife heard the sound of the LORD God as he was walking in the garden in the cool of the day, and they hid from the LORD God among the trees of the garden. But the LORD God called to the man, "Where are you?"

He answered, "I heard you in the garden, and I was afraid because I was naked; so I hid."

And he said, "Who told you that you were naked? Have you eaten from the tree that I commanded you not to eat from?"

The man said, "The woman you put here with me—she gave me some fruit from the tree, and I ate it." (vv. 1–12)

Truthfully, asking people to find the trauma is a trick question—one that exposes the reality of trauma. It's deeply personal, and deeply dependent on our individual values and perspectives. The trauma could be in any of the verses mentioned above, because trauma is different for everyone. What wounds one person may not even be noticed by another. Oftentimes we're drawn to investigate what specific parts of moments and experiences were traumatic, but the reality is, real trauma is the result of the experience, not the experience itself.

The experience causes the wound; the wound is the trauma that we live with.

With that in mind, what we *do* know is that in verse 6 of chapter 3, we see the wound. In Adam and Eve's perspective shift, we see the damage of doubt in God's goodness and their desire to protect themselves from it. But if we look back to Genesis 2:17, we see that God never said the tree was good for gaining wisdom; He said it was the Tree of Knowledge of Good and Evil. The lies of the Enemy wounded Eve's trust in God through manipulation, leading her to draw a conclusion that didn't reflect God's truth. When this happened, the wound of her heart became evident in her actions, and she ate of the forbidden tree.

The first trauma recorded in Scripture wasn't physical. It happened with words—I think it's important that we remember that.

> The experience causes the wound; the wound is the trauma that we live with.

THE INVERTED INTENTION

When we take a look at Genesis 3:1–12 from the moment Eve interacted with the Serpent, we see something interesting: the complete reversal of God's intention for humanity and their relationships with nature, themselves, and God. Adam and Eve once felt no shame toward themselves or each other. Now they were consumed by shame, as the creation they were trusted to care for became what they destroyed in order to cover themselves (v. 7). The closeness they felt toward each other dissolved as Adam addressed the "bone of my bones and flesh of my flesh" (2:23) as "the woman you put here." Eve, a gift from God to Adam in his loneliness, was now a burden to him, as he blamed her for their shortcoming. We even see this reflected in the different references for Adam's wife in Genesis 2:23 and Genesis 3:20. The "bone of my bones," whom Adam called "Isha" (woman) in the Hebrew, was renamed "Chava" (Eve) because of her role as mother to all. While her name prior to trauma was all about who she *was*, her post-trauma name was all about what she *did*. Most importantly, the trust God designed them to experience with Him was fractured by their fear of Him. The presence of God, the safest place they'd ever known, suddenly became terrifying. In the wake of trauma, the garden became a jungle, and the Priest became a predator.

The One who protected them from danger was now the One they sought to protect themselves from. What was once a clear understanding of who they were and who God was became disorganized and confusing.

Notice there is no joyful creativity in Genesis 3, because there is no space for creativity when you are consumed by fear. We see a great reversal of God's intention after Adam and Eve encountered the Enemy. Trust became mistrust, freedom became bondage, intimacy became burdening, safety with God became terror. Peace and belonging became shame and skepticism. Once, Adam and Eve had anticipated good things from God, but now they expected the worst.

This is what trauma does. It inverts the reality we were created for. Like Eve when she heard the lie that God was withholding, we assume the worst, fill in the gap, and draw conclusions that make us feel like we know how the story of our lives will end and how God will respond to our brokenness.

After Genesis 3:5, when the Enemy told Adam and Eve that their eyes would be opened if they ate the fruit, the Serpent disappeared. He never explicitly told them to eat the fruit. He simply asked the right questions to produce enough doubt in God's directive not to eat it. He sowed a seed of confusion and chaos in their hearts and vanished, leaving them with the wreckage of his manipulation.

In my clinical work, I've seen this time and time again. The workings of many of our traumas are so cunning, so complicated, and so inconspicuous that when we look back at the damage, we struggle to see the validity of our wounds. Rather than seeing our actions as a result of being manipulated or wounded, we see ourselves as inherently bad, as ones who did wrong things because *we* are wrong. In my opinion, I think this contributes to why so many trauma survivors struggle with suicidality. A client once told me, "If I am the problem, the only way to get rid of the problem is to get rid of me."

But you are not the problem. The way trauma has affected your life is the problem. The good news of the gospel is one where God restores all the intentions of Genesis 2 through the life, death, and resurrection of Jesus. The good news is that He will restore the original intentions of your life too. Adam and Eve's actions were an expression of the internal reality that came from their traumatic encounter with the Enemy. At one time, their thoughts, feelings, and actions reflected the original intention they were created for; after their trauma, their actions reflected the fear and shame of the lies they believed.

HEART TRANSFORMATION, NOT BEHAVIOR MODIFICATION

When we begin to allow God to shape and shift the perspective of our hearts, the patterns of our lives will follow. But this demands we dive into the dark corners that we've abandoned. If we want to change the fruit of our lives, we have to dig to the roots first.

I imagine that Adam and Eve, at some point, forgot they had lived with such unity and peace before encountering the serpent. Bombarded by the brokenness and destruction that trauma creates, I imagine it was hard for them to remember who they were before their world changed. I know that's true for me and for so many others. When enough bad things happen, we forget there was ever any good.

I know what it's like to hide from God as He calls out for me. In my shame, anger, and sadness, I expected God to be angry with me. I expected Him to chastise me, take away the things I loved, and take back the promises He spoke over me. The voices of pastors and spiritual leaders who preached that "grace runs out!" and "God is going to punish you if you don't _____" played over and over in my head. I was scared to be close to God and didn't feel safe or secure with Him.

But when I dared to surrender to His presence in the midst of my shame, I experienced something extraordinary—the very antithesis of the harsh and unmerciful words of people I'd listened to. My heart began to shift, and my mind began to think, feel, and act differently. It didn't happen overnight, but I was changing. I experienced God's tenderness. He did for me what He did for Adam and Eve in Genesis 3:21: "The LORD God made garments of skin for Adam and his wife and clothed them."

He covered my shame, rather than shaming me into not feeling it. He reminded me of my childlike joy and light. He reminded me of things that made me laugh. He gave me hope, and I began to want to live out of that instead of out of fear. As He ushered me back into secure intimacy with Him, I slowly but surely inched away from the fear-based connection I had with Him. He began to reorganize my perspective and bring clarity to who I was and who

He was—things that were once in complete disarray. When I was convinced that my life was defined by brokenness, God showed me that it was only derailed by it. There was a new path He was putting me on, and it would look like nothing I thought it could be. The traumatic experience of Adam and Eve shaped their world and ours too. It affected their patterns with themselves, each other, God, and the world they were called to steward. Trauma leaves no part of our lives untouched, distorting how we perceive ourselves and receive God's goodness.

But healing is possible. Restoration is possible. Redemption is possible. We have to discover and face what needs to be healed, restored, and redeemed. We have to open ourselves to the reality of the painful moments that fuel the unshakable patterns that keep us from the abundant life we were designed for. God can and will redeem the moments that shape the way we interact with the world around us. Becoming aware of our brokenness is the beginning of all healing. You can get your light back and experience what it's like to be your free, authentic self again, even if you don't remember ever being that self.

For Funmi, healing was being never deeply attached to people around her. It didn't include acknowledging her childhood or addressing the pain that made her want to bypass being in deep relationship with others. She came to discover that healing included going back further than she wanted but also going forward in a way she couldn't imagine. Funmi was initially unwavering about her desire to practice non-attachment. But when she became awakened to the wounds she carried and we began to work through the mental and emotional barriers she faced, she slowly became aware of the reality that her desire for non-attachment was a reflection of her fear and not of her heart's desire. Funmi got reacquainted with her desire to be in a safe and intimate relationship and developed skills to show up for herself in the ways her parents previously hadn't. Funmi began to find a sense of safety in connectedness within friendships she decided to reinvest in, and she recently got engaged to her boyfriend, who lavishes her with the attentive presence she's longed for since she was a child.

If we are going to dare to look at our wounds and how they affect us as we get out from behind the bushes, we have to allow ourselves to be seen in our brokenness, even if we can only bear to do it bit by bit.

Reflection Questions

1. What is one wound of the past that has changed your perspective of yourself, God, and/or others?
2. What changes did that wound make in the ways you interacted with others?
3. How did you interact with yourself, others, and God before you experienced that wound?

chapter two

NEGATIVE PATTERNS:
WHY CAN'T I CHANGE?

"Is it even possible for me to change?" Abena (Ah-bin-AH) asked with a sigh of desperation. "I feel like every time I try, I hit a wall, or something yanks me back to my old patterns. It feels impossible to try something new and stick with it. What is wrong with me?"

I could tell she'd asked herself that question many times, though it sounded like this was the first time she had said it out loud in front of another person. I leaned in, and her eyes lifted from the ground to meet mine.

"I can tell you're desperate for change, Abena, and you're reaching the end of your rope. I can also tell that you want change to come quickly." I let out a breath as I leaned in closer. "I have good news, and I have bad news. The good news is, the change you're looking for is absolutely possible, but the bad news is, it won't come quickly. But it can come. Hopefully we'll begin to see some beautiful changes as we explore some of your history. Together we'll gain understanding of some of the cycles you have that you don't like, and we'll begin working through those barriers."

She let out an exasperated groan. I could feel her frustration. Abena wanted change quickly. She wanted simple steps to help her get to the solutions that she was looking for. She wanted formulas, guarantees, or secret tips that would give her quick progress. But those things are Band-Aids, and soon she would come to discover that she needed something closer to surgery.

I learned a lot about Abena during our sessions together. She struggled with a lingering sense of inadequacy that she couldn't remember ever being free of. She thought she wasn't good enough, telling herself that she needed to just work harder to prove to others that she was intelligent and worthy of good things. These thoughts led to feelings of shame and anxiety that she would soothe by staying up late to watch a new television series with her favorite salty snack in hand. After a long night, when she'd wake up late the next morning, she'd struggle to meet her basic needs, like staying hydrated, eating balanced meals, and caring for her personal hygiene. She would feel frazzled at work from her rocky start to the day, leaving her overwhelmed by the time she got home. Ashamed of the mistakes she made at work because she was so unfocused, she would soothe that shame once again with a late night of binge-watching her latest series as she snacked the night away.

Abena dreamed of a life where she loved her body, ate what made her feel her best, and seized the day early as she worked on the business she dreamed of starting—an idea she'd had for years. But she felt trapped in the cycle of keeping up with life instead of living it. Her dysfunctional patterns made it hard for her to show up as her full self.

DETECTING DYSFUNCTION

All behavioral and thought patterns are results of repetition. *Dysfunctional patterns* are thoughts or actions that impair, disturb, or decrease our ability to maintain our overall health, connect to others, and live lives congruent with our personal values. When we repeatedly do or think things, it creates automatic circuits in our brain that cause us to engage in those behaviors with more frequency and less awareness.[1] Dysfunctional patterns are repetitive actions that contribute to our unhealth but also provide us a reward in some shape or form, making it hard to stop doing them.

In the creation narrative, we see Adam and Eve hide and cover themselves from God, easing their guilt and shame. Though that may have been a temporary reward, they failed to see how hiding distanced them from God. The garments that covered their shame were also barriers between them and God. Our patterns are our garments too. They allow us to be as close as we can tolerate, while covering the fear-filled wounds we've convinced ourselves we have to live with.

For many of us, the dysfunctional patterns we engage in reflect the values we absorbed from both the good and the bad experiences we've had. Constantly staying quiet when someone hurts your feelings or uses abusive language is a dysfunctional pattern that may reward you with a sense of safety in the moment by avoiding conflict, but it also contributes to your mental and emotional burden and normalizes an unhealthy belief that you're not worth protecting. Our dysfunctional patterns may also suppress our emotions when we get angry. In the moment, appearing calm may reward you with the appearance of maturity, but in the long run, it impairs your health by negatively affecting your heart health. A study done on the effects of anger on the heart found that suppressed anger was associated with death related to cardiac complications.[2] It's far too easy to forget that the price of staying silent is very real.

The cycle of dysfunctional patterns continues when thoughts produce feelings that affect our behaviors. When we change what we repeatedly think, we change how we repeatedly feel and behave. Our repetition shapes the physical structure of our brain, training it like a muscle toward healing and away from despair and destruction.[3] Maybe this is why Scripture tells us, "Whatever is noble, whatever is right, whatever is pure, whatever is lovely, whatever is admirable—if anything is excellent or praiseworthy—think about such things" (Philippians 4:8).

The dysfunctional patterns we engage in reflect the values we absorbed from both the good and the bad experiences we've had.

Our dysfunctional patterns are as diverse as we are. Some of our patterns appear in how we treat ourselves, and some of our patterns are most visible in our relationships with others. Though we desperately long for change, we snap at people after promising for years that we'll finally quit yelling. We tell ourselves we're going to stop disappearing into isolation when people hurt us, or that we'll finally speak up instead of shutting down. Show up instead of hiding, listen instead of being quick to speak, or speak up when we've been walked over for years. But the changes we want to embody don't stick. If we focus on the action of this cycle, we'll miss the opportunity to deal with the thoughts and emotions that often fuel them.

Some of us get stuck in cycles of incessant doing. We start new initiatives, explore new business ideas, and keep our days jam-packed with things to do. We are the ones gathering our friends, seeing needs, and then making plans to meet them. We start small groups, initiate book clubs, make the dinner plans, gather the recreational volleyball team, and check in on our friends, before we've checked in with ourselves. We say yes when we're worn down and exhausted, telling ourselves that one more thing won't hurt, especially if it's for a good cause. When we realize that our cups are empty and bone-dry, resentment rises as we feel used, unseen, and dehumanized by the people we once served with joy.

Dysfunctional patterns are repetitive actions that contribute to our unhealth but also provide us a reward in some shape or form, making it hard to stop doing them.

Sometimes we desperately long to be in the mix of life, going on trips, engaging in activities, and finally being seen by the people around us. But like chameleons, we blend into whatever background we are in, assimilating to whatever space we're in that day. We daydream of leading, speaking, and walking boldly as the person whom God created us to be. But the terrors of our past wounds tell us we aren't strong or good enough to live such lives. Our daydreams evaporate, and our pain becomes our only companion.

Like Abena, we are stuck in cycles of negative thoughts, feelings, and actions. These patterns are reflected in the ways we distract ourselves instead of engaging with the present, and in the ways we engage in negative self-talk as we internally berate ourselves for the things we do wrong. These patterns are displayed in cycles of watching porn, reading books to escape, overeating, avoiding confrontation, overdrinking, denying our needs, exploding into fits of rage, overworking, and defining ourselves by what we do.

It can be tempting to punish ourselves for being stuck in the cycle of negative thoughts, difficult emotions, and dysfunctional patterns. It's what so many of us do to ourselves because that's what's been done to us. We relate to ourselves the way we have been related to.

The ways that people react to our emotions and actions have taught us since birth how to regard ourselves and others. The ways that we care for ourselves are often an extension and reflection of how we've been cared for by others.

When we've had experiences that make us feel unworthy, unlovable, and undesirable, our automatic reaction is to turn our backs on those moments—to leave them in the past so we can move forward. We often express that moving forward as a reflection of faith—we are "moving on" and "not dwelling on the past." We think we're doing the right thing. All the while, we're feeding our shame and fear.

There's a difference between running toward something and running away from something, even if we're running in the same direction. The motive matters. If we're honest, we find that our patterns are often a reflection of running away from pain rather than running toward purpose. As long as our present actions are fueled by our past pain, our patterns won't change—not with sustainability and longevity.

Here is a core truth: We've been taught that our patterns are deliberate choices we make, when really, they're so much more.

They're responses to our experiences. If we want true change, we have to address the root of the problem instead of cutting off the branches. If we don't, the issues will just keep growing back.

THE NEUROBIOLOGY OF PATTERNS

Why is it so difficult for us to change our patterns? The biological answer is that our brains are wired to hold on to patterns as tightly as possible.

Our brains are made of neurological pathways that consist of neurons that are connected by dendrites. These neurological pathways are created by our actions and are strengthened by repetition. Every time we do something new, a new neurological pathway is formed. I think the odd, irritable sensation we feel when we're trying something new or learning something we don't understand is a reflection of that new neurological pathway being created. Discomfort can be evidence that we're doing something new.

The neural pathways created by our behaviors are the roads our brain uses to help our brain cells communicate with one another. This is called *neural firing*. Every thought, action, and feeling comes to fruition through neural firing. When the same brain cells connect over and over again, the process solidifies the existence of the road or pathway. Building powerful connections between the brain cells that create specific actions is often referred to as *wiring*.[4]

On a practical level, when we say over and over again that something is wrong with us, the repetition of those words strengthens the wiring of those ideas and beliefs in our minds. We can literally create paths in our brains that reflect specific thoughts we have about ourselves. Those thoughts then influence our behavior.

When we think a thought for the first time, that neurological pathway and the neurological network involved with that thought are like an old dirt path on grass. The more we engage in thoughts and actions that use that old, dusty path, the clearer that road gets. That means when we engage in thoughts and actions that validate our negative thoughts again and again, that old dirt road turns into a four-lane highway. We may start out with a few negative thoughts, but over time we begin to unconsciously speed down that highway of speaking poorly about ourselves, unaware that the constant repetition and wiring has made it neurologically easier to engage in those negative patterns. So much so that it becomes an uncontrolled, automatic behavior. For example: though it once may have been a less likely and difficult process to remain in abusive situations, the more we do it and the longer we endure it, the more we lose our ability to see what's abusive about the relationship at all.

Our patterns—our repetitive actions—are external manifestations of the thoughts and feelings we have internally. When we engage in these patterns frequently, they become automatic, like driving home when you planned to drive to the store or completing a task without even realizing you started it. These patterns can rule our lives, even when we don't want them to.

ABENA'S PATTERNS

Abena had been engaging in the same patterns for so long that she didn't even realize when she was in the midst of them, making them nearly impossible to stop. How can we prevent something we can't detect? We can't! And how can we stop when we do detect something, if we don't know what keeps it going? We can't!

Abena found herself noticing the cycle of automatic behaviors once they had already begun to negatively affect her life. She couldn't prevent them because she didn't understand what kept her in these patterns. She couldn't stop overeating, staying up late, or dropping the ball on work opportunities because she didn't realize in the moment she was doing it. When she did catch on to her destructive patterns, they'd already done so much damage. Frustrated with the state of her life, she made the mistake we all make at some point in our lives: we try to fix the outcome without addressing the root cause.

We oversimplify years of having our brains wired toward behaviors that keep us away from the lives we want to live. Book after book, podcast after podcast, seminar after seminar, Abena searched for new things to do so she could replace the patterns that kept her from the life she wanted to live. She would pray for hours, fast for days, and never miss a church service, thinking that stringent religious rituals would prove to God that she was worthy of attention and was ready for Him to change her heart and erase her problems.

She couldn't get close to God because He wasn't an advocate to help her, He was an audience she had to perform for. So she learned to engage with Him through patterns of performance she could never keep up. When she was tired, weary, and unable to pray powerful and elaborate prayers, she thought it'd be better not to bore God with her mediocrity. She'd draw away, not even considering that God would want to be around her just because she was His daughter.

Time after time Abena was disappointed. The rise of hope and motivation that inevitably crashed into desperation and self-hatred was exhausting. She felt like she was longing and yearning for a change that would never come. From what she could see, she was the problem—the common denominator. She was the reason why she couldn't have the life she longed for.

The question we often want to ask ourselves is, *How can I change?* But the question we actually need to ask ourselves is, *What situations wired me (and my brain) to respond this way?* The cycle is not the problem; what caused the cycle to exist is what needs to be investigated.

BENEATH THE PATTERNS

"Let's talk about your family," I said enthusiastically to Abena.

Her face twisted. "Why? What does that have to do with the changes I want to see?" she asked.

"Well, I think your family history, childhood experiences, and past relationships may play a role in the cycles you're struggling to break," I suggested.

Though she was reluctant, we began to discuss how she grew up in a family where she always felt pressured to portray an image of perfection even when her life was in shambles. "I think my parents cared more about looking good than our actually being okay," she told me in one session.

Abena shared more and more about a childhood where she wasn't taught the value of taking care of herself apart from what other people thought of her. When no one was around, she struggled to do simple things like eat when she was hungry, drink when she was thirsty, or use the bathroom when her bladder was full. She was always preparing for a performance. Because her value was in her utility, she had so little care for herself that she struggled to feel motivated by positive emotions. Painful emotions like shame, fear, anxiety, and embarrassment were necessary to motivate her to take actions, even positive ones.

In Abena's life, it was clear to see that childhood patterns followed her into adulthood. Strengthened with time and repetition, they had become as automatic as breathing. She wasn't making an active decision to devalue herself; the road was already paved. She simply couldn't see herself as worthy of having her needs met for *her* sake and not anyone else's. Her brain was so thoroughly trained to dismiss her needs that she was the last to find out she even had any.

During one session, Abena shared an instance where she desperately needed to go pee during an important church service. "It was the ordination of my uncle, and my dad was one of the people honoring and ordaining him. My family sat on the front row, which was a special place to sit at our church. I leaned over to tell my mom I really had to go pee. She told me I couldn't go because it would look bad if I got up and walked out on the front row.

"My bladder hurt so bad I started to tear up; I was only six years old. I was struggling to hold it. I didn't understand why my mom wouldn't just take me to the bathroom. As we talk more and more about my childhood, that memory keeps coming up, and I keep thinking about how I do that to myself now."

The patterns of our everyday lives reflect our deepest unaddressed wounds. When we seek to change the patterns, we miss the opportunity to explore how the patterns started in the first place. Abena already had neurological pathways that were strengthened over years. Trying to "do better" wouldn't enable her to change the strong wiring her brain had toward defending itself and soothing its pain through the patterns she desperately wanted to banish from her life. As a child, her experiences had wired her brain to dismiss her needs; her present patterns were an expression of that neurological wiring. Abena's story is reflected in many of ours. We want more of life, we yearn for it—we can see it, taste it, and feel it—but for some reason we just can't seem to let go of the dysfunctional behaviors that distance us from our dreams. Those behaviors keep us wondering if we'll ever live the life we want, while we blame ourselves for not being good or strong enough to change.

Our inability to change isn't our fault. The change we're looking for won't come from acquiring more knowledge on positive patterns to adopt. It won't come from waking up at 5:00 a.m., forcing ourselves to do more, and shaming ourselves when we do less.

It is our responsibility to look at the past moments that fuel our dysfunctional behaviors. Not because we need to be better for other people, not so that we can be more lovable to others, but so that we can live in the freedom Jesus died for us to have. You deserve to know what it feels like to live an abundant life so that you can take hold of every promise that has your name on it.

THE STORIES WE TELL OURSELVES

Abena began to feel that her dysfunctional patterns not only affected her perception of herself and her performance at work, but they also affected her closest friendships. I remember a hard session we had after a friendship that was developing suddenly came to a halt. A friend of hers shared her hurt and disappointment that Abena hadn't checked on her after the sudden death of her brother. Abena wept on the couch across from me with a grief that I know only comes from rejection and a desperate desire to connect with others.

"I don't know what's wrong with me. No one wants to be my friend. I wanted to reach out, but I just didn't know how. I'm a terrible friend." Abena's low self-esteem left her feeling like she had nothing to offer to those in pain. She struggled to sit with her own heavy emotions and felt useless when it came to sitting with others'. Her sadness quickly hardened into anger toward herself.

I leaned in with an empathic presence, knowing there was more that needed to come out.

"I deserve to be alone," she continued. "I literally can't do anything right. No wonder no one wants to be friends with me."

I could feel her words, and she meant every one. "Is that the story you tell yourself?" I asked quietly.

Her eyes shifted up. "What do you mean?"

"You're a terrible friend who deserves to be alone because you can't do anything right—is that the story you tell yourself?"

She took a second to think. "I mean . . . yeah, if I'm honest, today is definitely not the first time I thought that or said that about myself. So, yeah."

I explained to Abena that when we experience situations repeatedly, we extract from them what feels like a "truth" about ourselves and our lives. Our mind latches on to situations that validate the "truths" we've gleaned from these stories, further validating our mind's desire to tell ourselves these stories over and over again. This is how our brains are wired by the experiences we have. These stories matter because the stories we tell ourselves become the world we live in. The patterns we engage in are simply expressions of the stories we tell ourselves. The world we feel we live in is often a reflection of the things that have happened to us.

When asked what else she felt undeserving of, Abena shared that she felt undeserving of almost any good thing unless she worked for it. As we unpacked the story of her pain, we discovered a devastating narrative that had been told and retold in her heart— deep wounds from an emotionally absent mother had left Abena frantically searching for identity.

One of the things I do with my clients when they begin to discover the pain that has been hidden for so long is help them turn their newly revealed emotions into "I believe" statements. Abena shared several words that described how she felt about herself. Left by themselves, those words would just be a series of negative thoughts, but when I asked her to turn those words into an "I believe" statement, Abena's response was earth-shattering.

"So I want you to tell me in one sentence a new story about the same situation, using the three words you shared with me that stem from your relationship with your mom. You can start the story with the words 'I believe.'"

She took a moment to think. Her glance shifted all over the room as her eyes began to brim with tears. She blinked as one tear dropped. "I . . . I believe that I'm weak, incapable, and careless."

"And how do you think this affects how you interact with yourself and your friendships?"

"So I'm scared and . . . don't know how to show up consistently for myself or my friends."

"Can you put that together in one sentence?"

The room was thick with revelation and honesty—the atmosphere of open wounds.

"I believe that I'm weak, incapable, and careless, so I'm scared and don't know how to show up consistently for myself or my friends."

Abena had finally begun to see what lingered beneath the tip of the iceberg. Her patterns of withdrawing weren't moral failures or signs of laziness like she thought. They were perfectly sensible responses to the world around her based on what she had experienced in the past. Those experiences led her into the cognitive behavioral cycle of thinking she was weak, incapable, and careless; feeling inadequate; and then acting on the urge to withdraw and distract herself with late nights up and overeating to cope with those feelings of inadequacy.

Like Abena, many of us live in worlds that reflect the stories we've been telling ourselves for years. We engage in patterns we can't let go of, based on past experiences we've had that still linger in our present. Abena's everyday patterns were a reflection of how she could cope with painful thoughts and feelings related to her past.

Our dysfunctional patterns often help us cope with the difficult and complicated feelings we would have to address if we put them down and let them go. Beneath the surface of our everyday actions are unresolved feelings, narratives, and perspectives of ourselves that we would be forced to look at if we didn't have the patterns to distract us.

Most of us are largely unaware of how much our brain needs to hold on to these patterns to feel safe, even when they keep us from the abundant life we're longing for. There are things about ourselves, our abilities, and our worthiness that we believe to be true, and we can validate those beliefs with long lists of betrayals, heartbreaks, and suffering. We only identify patterns that don't give us the results we want.

When we don't have an awareness of our pasts and the patterns they create, we get stuck in pursuit of quick fixes, trying to create new habits while banishing others. Abena's limiting beliefs about herself and her habit of being absent in friendships was fueled by something that felt completely unrelated: her relationship with her mother. In that relationship, she had experienced emotional neglect and abandonment. The origin of her story was what she experienced growing up. Those past experiences created internal narratives that then created dysfunctional patterns in the present. The cold and unyielding story that she told herself lacked compassion and mirrored the words and posture her mother had toward her.

The story Abena began to discover in our sessions was one that saw her as human, wounded, deeply affected, and still worthy of love. But first she had to look deeper into past situations she didn't want to explore.

The stories we tell ourselves become the worlds we live in. When we can identify the stories we tell ourselves, we develop the ability to pause and take action to combat the narrative of the past and reflect the God-breathed narrative of the future. When hardship comes, when we don't get what we want, when we feel abandoned, betrayed, alone, or unworthy, these moments are invitations to identify the spaces that fuel our dysfunctional patterns. And when we locate these moments, we can trace our steps back to when those beliefs were first introduced to us (implicitly or explicitly) or when they felt most true in our lives. When we can define the moments that led to dysfunctional patterns, we have the opportunity to understand how those narratives affected us.

The stories we tell ourselves become the worlds we live in.

THE WOMAN AT THE WELL

When I think of Abena, I think of the Samaritan woman at the well in John 4. When that woman met Jesus, she was alone drawing water in the middle of the day, which was against the custom of her people, who drew water early in the morning, in groups. This was typically a communal outing for women in the community.

As the woman toiled alone in the heat, Jesus approached and

asked her for a drink, a simple gesture that redefined her world. As a Samaritan woman, she was considered unclean by the Jews. Jesus, the most Jewish of them all, never should have spoken to her, but in true Jesus form, He did what He wanted. As they continued to talk, Jesus asked her to go get her husband, and she denied having one. "The fact is," He said, "you have had five husbands, and the man you now have is not your husband. What you have just said is quite true," Jesus replied (v. 18).

When Jesus said this, I wonder what story this woman, who'd either been cast out by her community or had estranged herself from them, began to tell herself. I imagine she had been telling herself stories of how she deserved to be alone because of how many husbands she had, or maybe she told herself she didn't deserve love, which is why the man she was currently with was not her husband. Maybe she told herself stories of not deserving friendship or community. I bet she even told stories of not needing community or love at all, to guard her heart from the sting of rejection.

At the well, Jesus opened her heart to another story. But first He helped her see how her past experiences affected her present actions. He exposed the truth of where her heart was by bringing up her past as she stood alone in the heat. She was a woman who'd surely gone to the well many times alone, whose brain was wired to normalize loneliness and isolation, and Jesus came and interrupted her normal processing, stopping her from relaying quick and automatic actions of isolation in order to begin paving an old gravel road of intimacy.

As He simply sat with her, Jesus continued the process of renewing the woman's way of thinking and perceiving herself, the world around her, and the God before her. His complete and infinite love for her created a new way for her brain to process old paths and express new patterns.

John went on to tell us that the woman at the well lived in the new story Jesus told her. She developed courage to break her pattern of isolation and ran fast and hard toward community, relaying the intimacy she was given by Jesus. She told a whole town about a man who reminded her of her painful past but who changed the narrative she believed and lived in and who renewed the way she showed up in the world.

Like the woman at the well, Abena had corrective emotional experiences through therapy that changed her patterns from the inside out. In our time together, she began to receive the acceptance she had deeply craved from her mother and was even able to give it to herself. She began to listen to her body, take more breaks throughout the day, and meet her own needs regularly. She built routines of taking care of herself that were rooted in honoring who God created her to be, instead of how productive she could be. She rested often, had completely unplanned weekends, and found joy in her days instead of dread. Abena discovered a deep appreciation for herself and began to live a life fueled by an authentic desire to love herself and others.

What Jesus did for the woman at the well is what He is still doing every day for me, you, and Abena. He's unveiling the dark moments that make us feel least like who God calls us to be, to heal our hearts and redeem the past. Jesus sees you. He knows the complexity of the cycles and patterns you can't seem to shake or break; He knows the neurological, spiritual, and relational implications of them. Nothing has escaped His sight, not a wound or a tear. He looks at you with pride, joy, and hope as He calls you into the unknown territory of healing. He sees your despair, He feels your loneliness, and He is not taunting you with the dreams of your soul; instead, He is keeping them near as a reminder of how He will satisfy the desires of your heart with good things.

Change is coming, and change is here. It won't come from doing more; it will come from leaning in, from surrendering again and again and embracing your identity as a child of the Good Father.

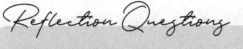

Reflection Questions

1. What is one dysfunctional pattern you have right now that you want to let go of?
2. What momentary reward does it give you?
3. What detrimental effects does it have on your life?
4. If, from this second on, you never got to engage in this pattern again, what emotion would you be forced to feel?

chapter three

CONFRONTING THE PAST: WHY CAN'T I ENJOY THE PRESENT?

When I was in college, I had a hard time confronting people who hurt me. I constantly avoided conflict until I absolutely had to deal with it. When someone said something hurtful, I lived in cycles of feeling wounded and talking to others about it but not wanting to address the person who actually hurt me. One day I spoke to my friend, who is now my brother-in-law, about it over lunch. As we chatted he asked me this question: "What do you do when a kid says there is a monster under their bed?"

I took a second to think about it. Finally I responded with enthusiasm, "Um, you tell them to come into your room and sleep with you!"

"Wrong," he replied. "You go into the room with them, and you tell them to point out the monster and tell it to leave. You encourage them to acknowledge the fear they feel, but you remind them that it's *their* room. *They* have control over it. If you let the monster chase them out of one room, it can chase them out of any room."

This conversation has become a parable I've told myself many times. It stuck with me. My brother-in-law was helping me see that if I avoided doing hard things to escape the fear I'd have to face, I would begin a pattern of allowing fear to control how I live and what I do.

In my work, I meet with clients who've spent their entire lives fleeing whenever there is a "monster" in the room—the monster of their past memories, conflicts, or chaos. They think a monster is after them. They feel like it's going to pop out at any moment. They act like one wrong move will draw it out of the darkness. When we live in fear, facing the scary things in our lives doesn't even feel like an option. When the monsters jump out of the closet, we simply leave the room, not noticing that most of our choices are driven by our avoidance of fear as we subtly allow it to become our master.

By the time I share this parable with my clients in our sessions, they can tell there's a monster in the room. They can identify the daily patterns they want to give up but just can't. The hope they have for the future is eclipsed by the pain and fear of the past. Somehow, they're at a crossroads, and the monster is in the room again. The self-sabotage has happened once again, the fragmented memory has returned, and the rage-filled outbursts and anxiety attacks have made their way to the front and center of their lives once more.

This chapter is for those who are ready to look back in order to move forward—those who are ready to recall and remember the things that fuel the destructive patterns of their lives. It's time to stay in the room. It's time to take the first step on the journey to healing: acknowledging the pain.

STAYING IN THE ROOM

In every season of my clinical work, I've had a client who's all but hunted me down for a session. I'm talking several emails a day, phone calls every week, and enough voice mails to fill a mailbox in a minute. Though it's not always fun getting so many forms of communication, my heart softens, because I can almost feel their desperation. They're thirsty for healing and simply can't go on living the way they have been. I know that feeling too well.

Esi (Ay-see) was one of those clients. Though my caseload was full, she waited three months to get on my calendar. She was relentless about her healing. So when she came in for a session one fall morning, I was ready to get to know her, hear her heart, and discover what she wanted help walking through.

During our first session Esi told me that she was anxious all the time, sharing that the only time she wasn't anxious was when she was depressed. As a young woman in her midtwenties, she was itching to really live life—to build meaningful friendships, to give love a shot, and to take risks in her career. But for some reason, she just couldn't.

"I feel like every time I try to build relationships, I get excited at the idea of being known and seen, but when I actually have to reach out to the person, I just can't do it. If we end up getting connected, I retreat into my shell. I wish I could be myself around people, but I just can't. I don't know why." The look on her face made it clear she had so much more to say. But her lips were pursed tight as her eyes shifted quickly from one end of the floor to the other.

Since it was our first session, we made our way through some preliminary questions, and I began to dive into her relationship with her family members. She'd told me about her close-knit family, which had experienced the same ups and downs that most families do: job losses, moves, and transitions.

As I asked about her relationship with her mother, sisters, and brothers, Esi lit up. She went on and on, sharing their childhood memories, bursting into laughter as she remembered the silly things they'd done and said together. She took a deep breath to punctuate her giggles, and she signaled that she was ready for the next question.

"What's your relationship like with your dad?" I asked. "What's your earliest memory with him?"

Esi froze. Her eyes shifted, and her body did all it could to curl up in a ball while staying seated. "It's good. We're fine. We've had some issues, but we're fine."

I tilted my head as I looked at her with compassion, leaving silence in the room for her to move in courage if she wanted to.

"You know what?" she said suddenly. "I don't even know why I'm here. I'm fine! I need to be grateful for the life I have. Maybe you can just help me develop more gratitude and a better perspective on life."

Her words were defensive, but her tone was frantic and terrified. The fiery excitement she had when she sought me out extinguished into smoke. I honored her unspoken boundaries, knowing we hadn't built enough trust for me to push, and we finished the session by talking about her work and educational history.

As I walked her to the door after scheduling our next appointment, she turned around, looking me in the eye for the first time. "How did you know to ask me about my earliest memory with my dad? You didn't ask about that with anyone else in my family."

I cracked a warm smile. "When you've experienced certain things, you know what questions to ask."

Her face softened. "I'll see you next week, Kobe." She quietly closed the door behind her. I could feel the embers burning.

I walked back to my chair, then sat with all the emotions Esi brought up for me. Though my father doesn't feature in my story of pain, not even a year prior I had sat in the exact spot she did, wrestling with my own truth.

LOOKING BACK TO MOVE FORWARD

In the fall of 2019, I sat in my brand-new counseling office in South Charlotte. It was a sanctuary of sorts for me. I often got there an hour or two before my first session to pray over the space, intercede for my clients, or drink a cup of coffee. Occasionally, God would speak a word that was specific to my personal life as I prayed. This was one of those days.

I had a complicated childhood, with what I struggle to call sexual abuse. I think inappropriate sexual touch would be the best phrase for it, but I know others might call it something else. And that's okay; our experiences are ours.

I remember being between four and five years old and seeing random commercials of people kissing, hugging, or rolling around in bedsheets (which I now know to be depictions of sex). I was never watching them outright but would catch a glimpse when one of the soap operas went on commercial break.

In 2017, while still in college, I began having vivid dreams of myself as a child, touching and inappropriately being touched by other kids my age. Scenes of us watching people kiss on TV shows and movies, then turning around to say, "Let's try *that*." These scenes haunted me for months. I would wake up nauseous, afraid, and ashamed. Somewhere deep in my heart I knew it wasn't just a dream, even though I desperately wanted it to be.

As a college student, I spoke to my campus minister about it. After many hard questions and even more tear-filled prayers, I finally had the courage to acknowledge that those moments weren't dreams, but memories of things that actually happened.

All of this was coming up again in 2019. God brought to mind one of the kids who was in my recurring dreams. I felt the Lord urging me to reach out and let them know that I remembered what happened when we were kids. In this instance, I recalled this individual touching me inappropriately. I was terrified. Did they remember? Was I making this up? What would they think of me?

I didn't want to reach out, but I knew that I had to. So, I literally held my breath as I called them and shared my memory with them as quickly as I could. They remembered too. They felt shame too. I could feel both of our burdens melt away as the truth came into the light.

The conversation was brief, heartfelt, and full of forgiveness on both ends. I felt proud of myself for facing my fear and experienced so much joy in knowing that neither of us had to carry this burden of secrecy and shame anymore. I reminded myself that this is what happens when we choose truth over fear.

A few months later, the memories started to happen again. Fragmented images flashed in my mind before I fell asleep, of my younger self initiating inappropriate touch with another child my age. I initially shooed them off as demonic attacks and tried to ignore them. But the images kept coming up at night and in the heart of the sweetest moments with God during my devotional time.

I could feel the Spirit tenderly hugging me, telling me that I wasn't defined by those moments. Something felt especially disturbing and heartbreaking about knowing that I'd initiated the inappropriate touch with another child. I was just a kid. I knew I didn't understand what was going on. Still, I was distraught. Every thought in my head screamed that I was a predator, a fraud for committing my life to helping others heal when I'd likely deeply wounded another person—all the while forgetting that I was deeply wounded myself.

I'm a terrible person, I thought to myself. *Nobody can know. What will people think of me? Will they trust the work I do?* I was scared. Certain that my actions as a five-year-old would define the rest of my life, I had promised never to tell anyone. But on that day, God told me to make the call to the person in the memory.

I protested for two days with tears of desperation. "God, I don't want to! Just make me forget again!" I wanted to run away from the truth. Hide and pretend it never happened. But what would that do to my soul? What would it do to the person He wanted me to talk to? God wanted this healed for a reason. He wanted me healed too. He wasn't trying to embarrass me or make me feel worthless. He was trying to restore broken things. He was giving me the gift of healing even when it didn't look like it.

I'd spent so many years praying for restoration, and this was how some of it was going to happen. The warmth He blanketed me with in my worst moments reminded me that this was God doing a good thing for everyone involved. Every tear I shed before the Lord was met with such warmth and kindness. He comforted me. He encouraged me.

What I didn't know was how much I'd truly need encouragement for what He was going to ask me to do next: call the kid I saw in the image and talk about what happened.

ACKNOWLEDGE THE PAST

The first step in facing the bogeyman of our past is acknowledging the painful moments. We have to turn our hearts toward the moments we've been taught to turn our backs on and look at those moments for what they are. We can't heal what we refuse to acknowledge. If we don't know where the bogeyman is, how can we tell it to leave? When we turn our hearts toward it, we have to speak about it.

Trauma therapist Diane Langberg said, "Trauma does not heal apart from being spoken, and it needs to be heard in the context of a safe relationship where the dignity of the one crushed is restored."[1] I didn't yet know it, but God was inviting me into that restoration through trusting Him in the painful process of acknowledging my trauma and speaking about it.

SPEAK ABOUT IT

The idea of having a direct conversation about something that brought me so much shame made me want to throw up. Still, something felt urgent, and I knew that, even though I didn't want to do it, if the One who comforted me through my shame was asking, maybe it was good for me to do. Though I wanted to do what God said, I found myself vacillating between telling myself I didn't need to make the call because everything that happened was in the past and nothing could change it, and telling myself that God can see more than I can so I should trust Him. I decided to go with the latter.

Over text I reached out to the individual and asked if they had a moment to take a call in the next few days. I told them it wasn't urgent and that I just wanted to chat with them. That Monday, I got to my office early to pray, thinking it would make me feel better, but it didn't. I remember saying out loud, "The fear isn't going anywhere; do it anyway," and with sweaty palms and pits, I found the contact of the person and pressed Call. The phone rang twice before they picked up.

After politely reconnecting, I started to share my feelings. "So I wanted to call to talk to you about something that's pretty sensitive. Are you in a place where you can hold that type of conversation? I'm nervous to talk about this, but the Lord has made it pretty clear that I need to have this conversation.

"God has been bringing up some things from my childhood that He wants to heal. And some of the instances He brought up were moments when we engaged in inappropriate touching. He specifically brought up moments where I initiated it." Tears were streaming down my face, but I knew I had to continue. "I just wanted to say I'm so sorry for hurting you, and I'm so, so sorry for the ways that it may affect you now as an adult. I want you to know that I remember and that I'm so sorry you experienced that."

There was a silence that felt like never-ending scratching on a chalkboard. I could feel their shock, anxiety, and even their relief. Finally they spoke. "I think about that moment all the time. I forgive you, and I don't blame you at all. We were just kids, and we didn't know what we were doing. I thought nobody remembered but me. I always thought something was wrong with me. I struggle with a porn addiction now and, honestly, I thought God was just fed up with me and gave up on me after all the times I just couldn't stop. Maybe this is a sign that He hasn't given up on me. Maybe this is a sign that He sees me."

We ended up speaking for about twenty more minutes as we comforted each other in our sadness of how that moment came to be and what it birthed in our lives as adults. We prayed for hope, healing, and restoration over each other through tears and comforting words.

Maybe this is a sign that He hasn't given up on me rang in my head for days. Before deciding to go through with the call, I had kept asking myself, *What good will this do?* After that call, I got to find out just how much good it *can* do when we stay in the room and face our monsters.

THE SCIENCE BEHIND CHILDHOOD TRAUMA

The things that happen to us in childhood, or any phase of life, don't dissolve with time. I think movies, media, and even religious systems can make us feel like if we just "press toward the mark," the ways we were wounded in the past will stop affecting us. But the truth is, we can't outrun pain. Whether we acknowledge it or not, we take it with us wherever we go.

Our childhood experiences are the very foundation of our understanding of the world we live in. They shape how we perceive ourselves and others, including God. They set the tone for who we believe we are and what we believe we are worthy of.

Our childhood trauma affects us more than just psychologically and emotionally; it affects us biologically as well, shifting the way our bodies operate, because our bodies are where these experiences are stored until we identify, address, and resolve them. The biological implications of the unhealed and unaddressed pain of our childhood creates the wiring of how our brains interact, which is the foundation of the patterns of our everyday lives.[2]

Between 1995 and 1997, Kaiser Permanente and the CDC conducted a study on 17,500 adults, investigating the effects of childhood abuse, neglect, and household challenges on the health and well-being of adults later on in their lives.[3] They named it the adverse childhood experiences (ACE) study. It measured the effects of childhood exposure to physical, emotional, or sexual abuse; physical or emotional neglect; parental mental illness; substance dependence; incarceration; parental separation or divorce; and domestic violence.

Each participant marked yes or no to an adverse childhood experience on the questionnaire. For each yes, the participant received a point. If a participant's parents were divorced, that counted as one adverse childhood experience. If the person's parents were divorced and their father sexually abused them, that was two points. If the person's parents were divorced, their father sexually abused them, and their mother was addicted to drugs or alcohol, that was three points. You can calculate your ACE score at the end of this chapter.

The results of the ACE survey showed that 67 percent of all adults had at least one adverse childhood experience. Incredibly, 12.5 percent of adults surveyed had four or more adverse childhood experiences. As scientists began to correlate ACE outcomes with health outcomes in adulthood, they discovered something shocking: the higher the ACE score, the worse the participant's health outcomes. A person with a score of four or more points on the survey was four-and-a-half times more likely to deal with depression, two-and-a-half times more likely to develop chronic obstructive pulmonary disease, and twelve times more likely to experience suicidality. A person who scored seven points or more on the ACE survey had three times the lifetime risk of developing lung cancer and three-and-a-half times the risk of ischemic heart disease—the number one cause of death in the United States.

The ACE study gave hard-and-fast evidence to the reality that we cannot outgrow our painful childhoods. We can't outwork them, outrun them, or simply assume that they no longer affect us because they were so long ago. No amount of ministry, philanthropy, or success can heal the wounds of our hearts that show up in our bodies, even if they were inflicted long ago.

Other studies have revealed that childhood trauma increases the risk of at least five out of the ten leading causes of death in the United States—heart disease, cancer, respiratory diseases, diabetes, and suicide. People who've experienced childhood trauma have a twenty-year decrease in life expectancy. When we've experienced persistent trauma or complex trauma, it affects our brain development, our immune system, and our hormonal system. It even changes our very DNA! What we don't resolve in our DNA is passed on when we have children, giving them biological disadvantages. When God allows our painful childhood trauma to reach the surface, and to find the light of day through being exposed in relationships, prayer, or therapy, He's not trying to torture us. He is not telling us to reenter the rooms where the most terrifying things happened to us because He wants to punish us. He's helping us reclaim the power, authority, peace, and freedom that we lost to the bogeyman of trauma. He's making us stay in the room because He's preserving our lives, as a good father does for his child.

PAIN CHANGES OUR BRAINS AND OUR LIVES

Within my first few sessions with clients who've experienced childhood trauma, they usually find a way to communicate that their pain isn't valid enough to hurt them as deeply as it does—especially my Christian clients. They'll go through a list of rehearsed statements when I begin to allow room for them to feel deeply about their experiences without my interrupting.

"It's not like I was sexually abused or something."

"I didn't have it as bad as others. I just need to get over it."

"But no one laid a hand on me."

As they continue to attempt to convince me of how their experiences really aren't that terrible, I think of all the times they must have been invalidated in the past. All the times they let their pain be seen, only for others to shame them into leaving it in the darkness. All the times they taught people how to dismiss their pain by dismissing it themselves so they wouldn't have to live with the unexpected sting of rejection.

Sometimes we'll turn our back on ourselves because we think others will, too, one of the most common acts of self-betrayal. I consider *self-betrayal* the act of denying or minimizing one's true nature, feelings, or needs in order to avoid conflict or judgment. It's a clever way to maintain connection with others and a quick way to lose connection with ourselves. Unfortunately, it's common for Christians to feel shame about their needs, because of how Scripture has been used against them. They often expect me to join the chorus of invalidating voices as they list off Bible verses people have used to shame them in the past. Instead, I lean in and listen. I stay right there, not letting the conversation move on. Whenever this happens, I think of those funny images of lazy dogs who are all but forced by their owners to go on walks. Rather than resisting or running back in the house, they just lie down, leash and collar attached, deciding they won't.

You don't have to be touched to be traumatized. The words spoken over you that sting to this day are evidence of that. The phrases that swirl in your mind, talking you out of trusting and risk-taking, are proof. Not thinking about the things you experienced doesn't mean the damage they've done in your life is gone; being hurt a long time ago doesn't mean you're not affected right now. You may think that what you went through was small, so you don't have to deal with it. I hear you. But you also know you can't keep living the way you have. The patterns of overdoing, underdoing, hiding, and craving the limelight have shoved you into the shadows of inauthenticity and shame. There's a reason God tells us to love our neighbors as ourselves (Matthew 22:39). We can't love others well until we love ourselves *first*. You may show up for yourself when people are watching, but how do you speak to yourself when no one can hear you? How do you treat yourself when no one can see you?

Deciding to "skip over" acknowledging and speaking about our trauma while trying to live a full and present life is like refusing to rehabilitate a sprained ankle to focus on running a marathon. Not only does it not make sense, but it's also incredibly dangerous. Similarly, deciding not to talk about your trauma or address it at all will cause incredible damage to your brain, body, and soul—the very things you need to live the life God has called you to.

Some of us don't feel worthy. We don't feel like we've been through enough to seek help or share our wounds. We feel like there's not enough shock and awe in our stories for people to care. After years of being told by parents, teachers, and pastors to "just let it go" or "leave it at the altar," seeds of self-loathing create the deep-rooted fear that our pain is still present because there is something fundamentally wrong with who we *are*. Your pain deserves to be seen, heard, and validated. No matter how big or small society says it is. You are not the problem. Your pain is; your wounds are. Being wounded doesn't make you a bad person. Being in pain doesn't make you a bad Christian. It means you need comfort and healing. You deserve to receive that.

The courage it takes to recall some of the worst moments of our lives is truly divine. It requires something outside of ourselves to revisit the times that made us feel like life was unsafe, scary, and not even worth living. But the harsh truth, from one trauma survivor to another, is that every time we don't look back and revisit the past to heal, we pay the price. Even when we're gifted, even when we're successful, even when we're "anointed." We don't have to live in the past. We don't have to be consumed by it. But in healing, we get the opportunity to look back at our past to process our pain and extract the wisdom that we need for our present. We can't move forward without looking back. I imagine that's why the word "remember" is used 253 times in Scripture. Remembering, confronting the truth of how we've been wounded, is what allows us to recover our lives from the trauma that's taken so much from us.

HOW LONG?

In Mark 9:14–24, a father brought his demon-possessed son to Jesus to be healed. No one had been able to heal him or help him. The first question Jesus asked this boy's father was, "How long has he been like this?" (v. 21).

I think Jesus wanted to bring to mind the full scope of this family's anguish. They needed to be fully aware of the size of their despair, so they could see that pain so deep and long-lasting can only have a divine solution.

I am not saying that your mental and emotional pain is a sign of demon possession. I *am* saying that Jesus asked this question because it matters how long we've been in pain. It matters how long we've been carrying these burdens.

In a similar way, God is calling you to remember how long you've carried your burdens so that you can become aware of how in need you are of His divine presence and healing.

Many of us have been wondering why the good moments of our lives don't stick. We don't understand why, even when our prayers are answered, we don't feel grateful or excited. We can't enjoy the present until we've made peace with the past. We have to look back; we have to stay in the room in order to heal.

Many of us learned how to be safe through hiding behind patterns. It's time to learn how to be free. We must face the things in the shadows and tell the bogeyman, "This is my house, and if anyone is leaving, it's you."

We can't enjoy the present until we've made peace with the past.

Reflection Questions

1. What situations do you feel God is calling you to acknowledge and talk about?
2. What emotions do those situations bring up? (Feel free to utilize the feeling wheel in Appendix B.)
3. Who is a safe and reliable person you can talk to? (A therapist is always a great option.)
4. When you feel the emotions a particular situation brings up, how do you cope with them?

Adverse Childhood Experiences (ACE) Study

The ACE questionnaire is a simple scoring system that attributes one point for each category of adverse childhood experience. The ten questions below each cover a different domain of trauma and refer to experiences that occurred prior to the age of eighteen.

Higher scores indicate increased exposure to trauma, which have been associated with a greater risk of negative consequences.

During your first 18 years of life:

1. Did a parent or other adult in the household **often or very often** . . . Swear at you, insult you, put you down, or humiliate you? **or** Act in a way that made you afraid that you might be physically hurt?   YES   NO   If yes, enter 1 _____

2. Did a parent or other adult in the household **often or very often** . . . Push, grab, slap, or throw something at you? **or** Ever hit you so hard that you had marks or were injured?   YES   NO   If yes, enter 1 _____

3. Did an adult or person at least five years older than you **ever** . . . Touch or fondle you or have you touch their body in a sexual way? **or** Attempt or actually have oral, anal, or vaginal intercourse with you?   YES   NO   If yes, enter 1 _____

4. Did you **often or very often** feel that . . . No one in your family loved you or thought you were important or special? **or** Your family didn't look out for each other, feel close to each other, or support each other?   YES   NO   If yes, enter 1 _____

5. Did you **often or very often** feel that . . . You didn't have enough to eat, had to wear dirty clothes, and had no one to protect you? **or** Your parents were too drunk or high to take care of you or take you to the doctor if you needed it?   YES   NO   If yes, enter 1 _____

6. Were your parents **ever** separated or divorced?　　YES　NO　If yes, enter 1
_____

7. Was your mother or stepmother: **Often or very often** pushed, grabbed, slapped, or had something thrown at her? **or** **Sometimes, often, or very often** kicked, bitten, hit with a fist, or hit with something hard? **or Ever** repeatedly hit at least a few minutes or threatened with a gun or knife?　　YES　NO　If yes, enter 1
_____

8. Did you live with anyone who was a problem drinker or alcoholic, or who used street drugs?　　YES　NO　If yes, enter 1
_____

9. Was a household member depressed or mentally ill, or did a household member attempt suicide?　　YES　NO　If yes, enter 1
_____

10. Did a household member go to prison?　　YES　NO　If yes, enter 1
_____

Now add up your "Yes" answers: _____. This is your ACE score.

Though any ACE score can negatively affect your overall health, scores over four are correlated to severe health risks and possible outcomes.

chapter four

FACING FEAR: WHY AM I SO AFRAID?

In her book *Trauma and Addiction*, Tian Dayton recounts a study that social psychologist James Pennebaker conducted on a college-aged student named Warren.[1]

Warren was a high-performing student. As valedictorian of his high school, he began his first year and a half of college strong. But seemingly out of nowhere, he developed anxiety. Halfway through the second semester of his sophomore year, he was stuck in a downward academic spiral, failing every single test that he took, which landed him on academic probation and forced him to later withdraw from school. For the next year, Warren went through therapy that sought to change his behavior and teach him relaxation techniques, but nothing was changing. His crippling anxiety was still there.

A year later Warren decided to visit psychologist James Pennebaker. Pennebaker agreed to talk to him about what was going on in his life under one condition: while Pennebaker spoke to him, Warren would wear a heart monitor to measure his heart rate as they talked about his life. The discovery made in these conversations was revealing.

When Warren spoke about his girlfriend, his heart rate was at 77 beats per minute, and he shared that he had some concerns about disagreements they were having. When he spoke about his college courses, his resting heart rate was 71, and he shared that most of his classes were actually interesting to him even though he'd been struggling with tests. When he discussed failing his exams, his resting heart rate was at 76, as he shared that it was "hard on his ego."

Things took a shift when Warren discussed his parents with Pennebaker: his heart rate rose to 84. He shared that they were a close family before his parents' divorce. When Warren explicitly spoke about the divorce, his heart rate increased to 103 beats per minute.

When asked to describe his parents' divorce, Warren said, "It was no big deal." But when he saw the results of how each conversation topic affected his heart rate, he was shocked. Apparently, it *was* a big deal! It was absolutely clear based on the heart rate monitor that the divorce was the source of Warren's stress and anxiety, even though he couldn't cognitively label it.

In the words of Pennebaker, "His body held what his mind disowned."

Warren carried the emotional and psychological pain of the past in the present, in a way seemingly unrelated to the behaviors he was trying to change. Many of us just want to learn how to relax, be less stressed, and focus more on areas that are affected by our deepest traumas. But sometimes, those aren't the actual issues that need to be addressed. The distress Warren's body had remembered about his parents' divorce left him anxious, with few ways to cope with the crippling anxiety. It made him believe he wasn't good at something he actually enjoyed and made him think he was unbothered by something that was ravaging his life.

This is what trauma does. It creates disorganized internal perspectives, affecting the way we understand ourselves and the world around us. The confusion it creates traps us in webs of fear and anxiety as we struggle to trace where one starts and another ends. All the studying in the world would have done nothing for Warren and his grades. School wasn't the issue, though it was affected. The deep pain he experienced from his parents' divorce was at the core of his anxiety. Without listening to his body, he never would have known.

Terror is defined as a state of intense or overwhelming fear.[2] But what does it look like to live with terror? It looks like being the valedictorian, acing every test but having a heart rate of 103. It looks like patterns that are destructive and need to be changed and also having patterns that are validated and praised. The unaddressed pain in Warren's life created patterns of success. Until they didn't.

Like Warren, many of us want to address the areas that are affected by our deepest traumas but aren't the actual issues that need to be addressed. We want to fix what is wrong on the surface without addressing everything happening inside us. But healing doesn't work that way. Esi came to learn this as we continued our sessions together.

FACING THE FEAR

After months of weekly sessions, Esi finally faced the heartbreaking reality that haunted her daily. A truth that made it hard for her to be seen and loved for who she was. She had constructed and lived as a version of herself that everyone saw but nobody knew.

During one session, after discussing that there was a "why" behind the things in her life that wouldn't change, she finally got the courage to share what happened to her. Through tears, trembles, whimpers, and wails, Esi strung together words she had never said aloud: "My father molested me for most of my childhood."

The confusing relationship she had with her father left her in a constant state of fear she didn't realize. She was terrified of speaking up for herself and even more scared of being seen and known by others, because it reminded her of the key features of the most painful relationship she had. She was his favorite child, she got extra attention, love, and affection, but she knew what her father did to her was wrong. She didn't like it but didn't know how to communicate that at such a young age.

When she got old enough, she distanced herself from her father with acts of defiance and rebellion. Though it caused him to stop abusing her, she also lost the fatherly affection she longed for. She wanted to tell someone but couldn't bring herself to do it. Esi pushed through life with a constant fear that rumbled under the surface.

Is it my fault that this happened?
Should I tell Mom?
Did he do it to any other children?
What would people think if they knew?

She threw herself into being the best at whatever she did. She was class president of her high school, graduated top of her class in college, got the job of her dreams after graduating, and led a Bible study for several years.

But she couldn't feel settled in her life or in her relationship with God. There was no peace, no matter how hard she sought it out. She couldn't live out of the joy and spontaneity that comes from freedom, because she was always preoccupied with presenting perfection. No one could see how shattered she was underneath it all. She saw God and Jesus as master and dictator and hesitated to step into the calling of "child of God" and "friend." She struggled to be honest in friendships for fear that someone would catch on to why she was estranged from her father, so she was always lonely. There was happiness from moment to moment, but it was always fleeting.

Esi had visitors in her life, but never residents. She had no joy, no freedom, no creativity, no spontaneity. Why? Because those things can't exist among fear; they certainly can't exist among terror.

The sense of terror we experience is one of the first things we face when we try to make small changes but feel great resistance. Like Warren, we know something is wrong, but we just can't name it. That doesn't mean we don't live with it. Our patterns become hard to let go of because they become our safety, the little bit of predictability in our confusing, disorganized, and terrifying lives.

When we stop binge-watching TV, overeating, isolating, or striving toward goal after goal, we are forced to face the loss of the things that comfort us and the reality of why we needed to be comforted in the first place. Terror often doesn't look like terror. It may look like laziness to some. It would have been easy to label Warren's swift academic decline as such. Our terror may also look like being really particular about certain things, such as having an intense dislike of something we can't explain or having an insatiable desire to have something or be loved by some type of person. Terror may look like being extremely tired all the time as you cope with triggers by sleeping. It may look like never wanting to rest for fear of having a still moment where painful emotions can rise to the surface.

The terrible experiences we've had create a pervasive sense of extreme fear that never really goes away until we look at what wounds us and get in touch with the thoughts, feelings, and perspectives we adopted from those wounds. Without that acknowledgement, our fear simply finds discreet places to express itself. For many of us, those places are in the ways we can't stop yelling at our kids even when we promise to, or the little white lies we tell to protect ourselves from the anger of those around us. They show up in the seemingly insignificant ways we go about our days, which makes it hard to define as *terror*.

Who wants to share that they're afraid, let alone terrified? Yet even when we don't admit it, it's still there.

A STARTING PLACE

Almost none of my clients come in saying, "I have trauma, I live in a constant state of fear, and I really want to work through it." Most of them come in saying things like:

"I just can't stop doing _____, and I don't know why."
"Every time I start doing _____, I go right back to what I did before."
"I just feel sad all the time."
"I can't stop crying."
"I think I have anxiety."
"I have trouble sleeping."
"I feel like my emotions are everywhere."
"I keep thinking about this, and I just want to be over it."
"I'm lonely but don't know how to connect."
"I keep sabotaging my relationships."
"There's so much I want to do in life; I just can't do it."

My clients are trying to find their way back to their authentic selves, but often through behavior change and not the restoration and healing of their minds, bodies, and souls. Wholistic healing that addresses the ways our trauma affects our whole selves allows new actions to be an outpouring of the new truths we hold dear, rather than actions we take to cope with pain.

These clients know the lives they live don't reflect who they *really* are. Each of those statements is a desperate plea to reclaim what trauma took from them: the sense of security, the sense of peace, the sense of assurance, and the belief that they are worthy of good things. Some of us don't even realize that we're trying to reclaim our authentic selves. We just know that something has to give, something has to change.

We have to walk down some dark roads to get to the light we were meant to live in. Still, we are worth it. Jesus' sacrifice for us is evidence of that.

Esi came to therapy wanting to understand why she wasn't close to others. She wanted a simple fix: teach me how to stop being afraid so I can be close to people. You may have the same posture: teach me how to change my patterns, so I can be more connected, creative, and spontaneous.

To that I say, *Let's start the journey.*

Terror freezes us in the traumatizing moments we haven't yet looked at or processed. To process trauma is to investigate the wounding thoughts, feelings, and perspectives we've developed about ourselves and the world around us. Processing our pain includes discovering what we needed but didn't get, so that we can discover what we need to give to ourselves in order to heal those past wounds and feel safe in our present experience of life. Without processing our trauma, we are stuck living in the fear of that moment even when we're not cognitively aware of it. It leads us to cycles of self-betrayal, self-sabotage, of engaging then withdrawing, and so much more.

Fear is a defining factor of trauma because it's the state our brains and bodies are stuck in until we address it. Am I saying you're living your life cowering in a corner? Not necessarily physically, but you might be emotionally. I think of it as one of those jack-in-the-box toys. You know a clown is going to pop out at some point, but you don't know when. Even though it may not have popped out yet, you're bracing for the moment when it will. If you've been wondering why you can't live the life you know you're called to, it's possibly because your life is driven by a sense of terror related to your trauma. You're trying to live well, but you're also terrified of that clown popping up at any moment—terror affects just about everything you think and do.

> To process trauma is to investigate the wounding thoughts, feelings, and perspectives we've developed about ourselves and the world around us.

TWO SIDES OF THE SAME COIN

Terror will convince you that the most wounded version of yourself is who you are. Let me tell you right now, it is not.

Being frozen in terror sometimes looks like quickly reverting to the scared person we were when we were first wounded, or having an inability to respond in ways that reflect our current age when faced with situations that resemble the environments that were so frightening to us.

If we're honest, we've all been surprised by how sad, angry, or fearful we've become in situations that on the surface seemed mundane. The child in us that never got to grow up made an appearance without our permission. And that child won't ever grow up until they get what they need. However, rather than meeting those needs, we shun the idea of childlikeness and deny ourselves the things we need to feel safe, doing to ourselves what others have done to us.

We live with the armor of performance in order to protect ourselves from being seen as the terrified people that we are. When all our energy is spent fiercely defending the image of ourselves that makes us feel safe, we don't have time for anything else. We have just enough to survive.

When our brain can make sense of everyday painful events, it operates with a sense of integration, which allows for some chaos or spontaneity and some rigidity or order. When our brain can't make sense of the difficult things we've experienced, it stores these moments as trauma and sends our brain into patterns of deep chaos or intense rigidity, missing the balance of the middle.

When we operate through a lens of chaos, we abandon all order and engage in behaviors that are erratic, adrenaline-seeking, and unpredictable. When we operate out of rigidity, we walk the tightrope of perfection, always making sure every hair is in place and breaking down if the slightest change affects our sense of order. Both of these postures are responses to not getting what was needed when it was needed. One person says, "I'll throw myself into harm's way to avoid being affected by hardship, since life can't be predicted anyway," and another may say, "If I had been in control, this would not have happened, and I need to control all I can to make sure it never happens again."

WHAT WE DO WITH THE TERROR

When we realize that we are operating in patterns of fear and shame, the greatest gift we can receive is the ability to feel safe. Trauma healing requires learning, courage, trust, innovation, imagination, and spontaneity. But the part of our brain that is activated when we are fearful and shameful shuts off our ability to learn and connect. Deep in our temporal lobe is an almond-shaped cluster of neurons called the *amygdala*, the emotional center of the brain.[3] When we are fearful, our amygdala is incredibly active, but the more our amygdala is activated, the less we are able to learn and connect with others. Without the sense of safety that allows us to learn or connect, we'll be stuck in the emotional cycles of fear and shame. There are several ways to begin to cultivate environments of safety within ourselves as we address our terror and increase our capacity for learning, connecting, and healing. Each of these methods of creating safety is deeply rooted in God's beautifully intricate biological design of humans.

Movement

The amygdala is a part of a greater system called the *limbic system*. The limbic system is responsible for behavioral and emotional responses, especially those related to our survival. When our limbic system is activated, we can calm that activation by telling it to decrease activity. We communicate with the limbic system through movement.

Movement allows us to decrease the activity of this area of the brain so that we can direct the body from being fearfully on guard to safe and calm. Movements like walking, stretching, dancing, and even shaking to release tension decrease the activation of this system, allowing us to feel safe in our bodies. It also allows the brain to absorb and retain the information needed for the healing journey. Without the biological sense of safety, we shut off our ability to experience emotional and spiritual safety. Healing happens in our bodies. Movement should always be a part of the healing journey.

Deep Breathing

Another way that we can access biological safety is through deep breathing. When we shift the way we breathe, we can shift the way our bodies respond. When we are anxious and afraid, we tend to have shallow breathing that is reflected in the rise and fall of our chest. This is the physical indicator that our sympathetic nervous system, which is responsible for our fearful trauma responses, is activated.[4] When we are rested and calm, our breath is centered in our belly and marked by the expansion and contraction of our stomachs.

Try this quick exercise: Breathe in through your nose for four counts, then hold at the top of your breath for two counts. Then exhale for six counts, breathing slowly through your nose. As you do this, imagine that your stomach is expanding like a balloon as you inhale and deflating as you exhale. Set a quick timer and do this for forty-five seconds.[5] This is one of the many deep-breathing exercises that can calm our body's fear responses and help us feel safe in our body.

The process of creating a sense of physiological calm, so that we can learn and connect, can be as simple as shifting how we breathe.

With breath God created new and good realities; in His likeness, He designed us to do the same. The intricacy and intentionality of God's design of the human body is absolutely fascinating. Truly, we are "fearfully and wonderfully made" (Psalm 139:14).

Safe Place

Safe Place is one of my favorite activities to utilize with my clients as we begin the journey of trauma healing. This activity is adapted from the beginning phases of a trauma therapy called Eye Movement Desensitization and Reprocessing (EMDR), which I often utilize with clients.[6]

The objective of Safe Place is to help you access feelings of peace, safety, and even joy despite your current distressing reality. When we think about places we love and feel safe in, we can access emotions in the present that are related to the past experiences we've had in those places. For someone who loves the beach, simply thinking about the sound of the crashing waves, the sensation of the wind on their skin, and the warmth of the sun can lead them to presently feel in their bodies emotions and sensations related to past positive memories at the beach. God created beautiful biological benefits to imagination, which we have access to as we heal. In this activity, answer the following questions:

- Where is a place, or what experience have you had, where you felt calm and/or safe?
- What does that place look like? Get as detailed as possible with colors, textures, and placement of items.
- What smells, sensations, sounds, textures, and temperatures do you experience in that place?
- What emotions do you feel in that place?

Now take a moment to close your eyes and envision this place with the positive emotions that it brings to you. As you imagine, notice where in your body those positive emotions present themselves.

When you've finished imagining and envisioning this place, write down what you saw, felt, heard, and smelled, along with the emotions and physical sensations you felt. After writing these down, go back to your safe space. Once you notice the physical sensations that are connected to positive feelings of safety and joy, cross your arms over your chest, with each hand touching right below the opposite shoulder. Slowly count to ten as you alternate tapping each hand below each shoulder.

This is a practice called *tapping*, a type of bilateral stimulation (stimulations on both sides of your body). Slow bilateral stimulation is a natural way we can consolidate or save memories, thoughts, and emotional sensations.[7] It activates both parts of the brain, which are needed for wholistic processing. The left side of the brain processes the "what" of how we feel, while the right side of the brain processes the "how." Tapping has several benefits, like calming our nervous system, and it adds a biological bookmark to what we are focusing on. With that bookmark, we can quickly access what we added slow bilateral stimulation to.

The first few times you try to access the images and sensations related to your safe place, you may need to open your eyes to read the descriptions and remember them. But as you add bilateral stimulation (always once you feel the positive emotions and sensations), there will come a time when you can simply name the place (i.e., beach, home), and your brain will flood your mind and body with all the images and sensations of your safe place. This is a great resource for people who experience frequent triggers, social anxiety, panic attacks, and the other manifestations of the terror our trauma creates.

LEANING IN

When we feel safe, we have the freedom to get curious about our experiences and our reactions. We gain the opportunity to really lean in to what our fear is communicating to us rather than become stuck in disorienting cycles of being controlled by it. Every thought and feeling we have has a story to tell us. When we are safe, we can listen. We can lean in to the stories we tell ourselves rather than distract ourselves from them.

Try as we might, we can't outwork the terror. No awards or accolades will make it go away. No shaming will change the biological reality we carry in our fear. We can't run away from it. It lives in our bodies and goes wherever we go.

The good news is that we can heal, even in the face of trauma and terror, when we dare to give ourselves the gifts of safety and rest *before* we feel like we've deserved it. That may look like taking a break from going to certain places, interacting with certain people, or doing certain things, to allow yourself to experience a level of safety. Meeting other people's expectations of what you should or shouldn't be able to do regardless of what you've experienced is not going to help you heal. Nor will pushing yourself to keep doing things that make you feel fearful, anxious, and shameful. Giving yourself tenderness, mercy, and safety will.

As I continued to work with Esi, she began to develop compassion for herself. She gained an understanding of the complexities of her experiences and realized just how freeing it was to walk through this process with someone who could support and empathize with her without judging her. She realized she didn't have to take this journey alone. She allowed herself to feel deeply without shame and faced the truth of her pain. She began to see that, although her abuse deeply affected her, it didn't define her.

Without the pain of her secret holding her down, she began to see in other people the signs of sadness, loneliness, and despair that she herself lived through. She felt hope for the first time in years as we processed the wholistic effects of her childhood abuse. She felt empowered to love again and to allow herself to be loved. Because of the healing she experienced in therapy, she decided to pursue a degree in Christian counseling. I have the honor of knowing her as a colleague in the field today. The life you want to live is possible. The joy you want to know is real. Your momentary fear is normal; your terror is not. Your armor is cracking because it's time for healing; it's time for the abundant life you dreamed of—a life made for the *real* you. In the safety of being released from the grip of terror, your most authentic self can breathe deeply, even if it's just for a moment. The truest version of yourself can be tended to, understood, and healed. There is triumph beyond the terror.

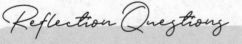

Reflection Questions

1. How does my terror present itself in my life behaviorally? What things do I struggle to let go of?
2. How do I act when I don't feel safe?
3. What do I feel when I do feel safe? What do I imagine safety feels like? Where does that show up in my body?
4. Take time to utilize one of the safety techniques we reviewed earlier. Make sure to journal what your experience was like.

chapter five

INVESTIGATING IDENTITY: WHY IS IT SO HARD TO LOVE MYSELF?

For years, I believed I was bad. Every action I took was in pursuit of silencing the voices in my head that told me that I wasn't worthy of love unless I was striving. This belief led me to live out patterns of self-betrayal in both big and small ways. I struggled to speak up when something unjust was done to me. I talked myself out of getting my basic needs met as they arose, telling myself *I'll eat after I finish this,* and *I'll go to the bathroom after one more task on my to-do list is done.* The little moments of my life were littered with evidence that I didn't deserve the simplest of things unless I earned them in one way or another. I was bad. Therefore, all good things had to be earned.

I believed that if I stopped my patterns of self-abandonment and self-betrayal, I'd also be stopping the only way I could get love. I needed love, so I always found my way back to my destructive patterns. I still desperately needed those unhealthy patterns I wanted to break in order to invalidate the lies I'd come to believe about myself through the traumas I'd experienced.

The lie—*I am bad*—was my negative core belief. This lie shaped my perception of my identity and my perception of the world. I couldn't confront this pattern until I felt safe enough to peel back the layers of coping and distracting, to discover the driving force of my most mundane actions.

A *negative core belief* is a lie about our identity and worthiness that we believe to be true, even when we don't want to. These core beliefs about our identity are explicitly or implicitly communicated to us through the traumatic experiences we have. For example, a child who has a parent that is only attuned to their needs when they succeed may have the negative core belief, *I am worthy of love only if I earn it* or *I am unlovable without accolades.*

Sometimes negative core beliefs are a product of specific moments, and other times they are reflections of several different instances that create a common negative feeling or perception of ourselves, leading us to adopt a lie that makes sense of the many painful experiences we have. For example, a child who had emotionally unavailable parents may develop a negative core belief that they are unlovable. A child who was always made to be responsible for their caretaker's emotions may have a negative core belief that states, *I am not good enough* or *I'm responsible for all bad things that happen.* The expectations we put on ourselves reflect what we believe about ourselves. If we constantly feel the need to do something for someone before we ask something of them, we may silently believe that we are not worthy of love unless we provide value to another person first. If we feel like we need to always be excited or in a good mood to spend time with a friend, we may quietly believe that people will only love one version of us or that we only deserve good things when we feel good. These small relational patterns that arise when we don't feel like our best selves create bread crumbs that lead to the truth of what we believe about ourselves.

If we believe we are worthless, we're less likely to allow people to sacrifice for us, or, in turn, to sacrifice for them, since we feel we have nothing good to offer. When we believe that we're alone, we're constantly anticipating people's departures and more likely to interpret their unsavory qualities as evidence they are going to abandon us at any moment, rather than it being a reflection of their bad day. In these cases, our lives feel disorganized and confusing as we flip-flop between living in the past and living in the present.

THEY ARE LIES

The first time Kidist (Ki-dist) came to see me, she bluntly asked at the end of our session, "Why am I like this?" She didn't understand why she couldn't stop committing to things that drained her. She had a compulsive need to sacrifice for the people in her life but didn't know why she couldn't give herself what she needed and set boundaries that allowed for rest and downtime.

I took a breath before I responded to her. "I think there are some deep wounds that are keeping you from loving yourself the way you need and desire."

She stared blankly. She knew what I said had the familiar ring of truth, but her hope was to change her patterns, not to explore them. She wasn't initially interested in following each action from the fruit of behavior to the root of her heart's posture. She didn't want to go there. But the freedom she was looking for was buried in the soil of her heart, and she wouldn't see freedom until we got to digging.

Negative core beliefs are the result of deep wounds. They are the infected, bacteria-filled wounds that affect how we function. They are lies. No matter how true our negative core beliefs feel, they are *always* untrue. They make us feel like our temporary experiences reflect our permanent values and that our permanent identity in Christ is temporary.

THE VICIOUS CYCLE OF LONELINESS

Without our even realizing it, our negative core beliefs can leave us in loops of *reenacting* the moments that made us feel worst about ourselves. These reenactments are relationship dynamics that are constantly re-created in our lives as they seem to follow us in and out of season.

I once had a client who had the negative core belief "I am toxic." He believed that if people stayed with/around him too long, he would hurt them. That negative core belief showed up in his friendships, where he experienced deep intimacy, then, out of nowhere, found a way to sabotage the relationship. He would be an incredibly kind and generous person as he got to know the person, then unexpectedly became cold and distant, saying mean and hurtful things to someone he genuinely liked. For years, he unconsciously "warned people" with his unexpected, cold behavior to not get too close, even when he wanted them to be. Growing up, he had parents who often emphasized his responsibility in anything that went wrong in his life. Even when he was victimized by others, his parents always shared what he "could" have done to prevent himself from being hurt by others. Over time, he grew to believe he was toxic and all the pain in his life was his fault. Though he longed for intimacy with others, his self-sabotaging behaviors scared people away like a hazard label on harmful household chemicals.

The relational patterns we constantly experience point to the traumas we've endured. The person who struggles to feel close to God after experiencing spiritual abuse may find themselves avoiding intimacy with God by believing they already know what God is going to say or how He is going to respond to them. Their actions keep them distant from Him as they try to protect themselves from feeling abandoned by Him. But when they guard themselves by trying to beat God to the punch of rejecting them, they leave themselves isolated from His love.

The lies we believe about ourselves and the world around us cause us to engage in *transference*, which is placing the weight of a past incident on a present moment.[1] We treat the people who forgot to show up for us once like the people who didn't show up for us for years. We may find ourselves saying, "You always do this!" to someone who has only let us down once. Even though we're talking to the person in front of us, we're really responding to the ghosts of our past.

When we are stuck in cycles of reenactment and transference, there's no space for authentic connection. Not with ourselves. Not with others. Our romantic partners become people reauditioning for the roles that others previously failed to perform well in, and our children become new opportunities to correct the moments we haven't dealt with, instead of being sacred people who bear the image of God in a unique way. Each person becomes a prop in the story we are trying to unconsciously rewrite. When that happens, they can only be seen and regarded through the pain we've endured.

These lies, these negative core beliefs that distort how we see ourselves, the world, and our relationships, often lead to *ruptures*, the painful deterioration of our deepest relationships. A rupture is a disconnection in our relationships with others.[2] These disconnections can happen through feeling unseen, being dismissed, having arguments, or struggling to feel close to others. At its core, a rupture is a loss of trust and safety. Something many of us are all too familiar with due to the traumas we've experienced. If you've ever felt the need to distance yourself from a friend after a conversation in which they said something that made you feel uncomfortable, you've experienced a rupture. If you've been skeptical about attending a church after discovering how downright mean, discriminatory, and graceless your previous church was, you've experienced a rupture. If you constantly need to double-check your partner to make sure they follow through with their promises, you've experienced a rupture.

The relational patterns we constantly experience point to the traumas we've endured.

Everyone experiences ruptures in relationships, but not everyone recovers from them. When we feel safe, we view ruptures through the lens of curiosity and a desire to learn and gain mutual understanding. When we're in a state of fear, we view ruptures as personal attacks or threats of abandonment. We can become defensive and attack back—the fight response—or do whatever we possibly can to regain safety and security in the relationship, at the expense of our feelings, truth, and perspective—the fawn response.

This is the vicious cycle of loneliness. The negative core beliefs we unconsciously live through lead us to seek out relationships with others only to reenact and transfer our past unresolved issues onto the people we are seeking to connect with. As we wrestle with the ghosts of our past in the people of our present, we experience ruptures that then lead us back into social, emotional, and spiritual isolation. When that isolation gets unbearable, we find ourselves seeking out new sources of connection, only for the cycle to begin again. The core of the cycle is our unresolved trauma—the lies we believe about ourselves because of what we've experienced.

Negative core beliefs trick us into not believing that we are who God says we are. They create conditions in our heart that make it hard to love ourselves, others, and God. The lack of safety we feel in the world leads us to connect through fear and shame instead of joy and authenticity. These lies keep our eyes ever fixed on the terror of the past, causing us to forfeit the gift of hope in the future.

When I tell my clients that their negative core belief is a lie, they almost always take on a lawyerlike defense. I remember one client saying, "Well, all evidence points to the fact that this lie is true." We both chuckled, but even in her joke was a resolve that her internal lie of being unlovable was true.

"Is it true?" I asked. "Or is it all you can see?"

Identifying a negative core belief with a client is often a heartbreaking moment. A time when their wordless groans find language, and hidden wounds touch fresh air. We can begin the process of moving toward freedom when we expose the lies we believe to new environments and new voices. We have to break the mold of what we do, whom we interact with, and how we engage, in order to challenge these lies and expose ourselves to experiences that reflect something other than what we currently feel. This is why creativity and spontaneity are at the core of all healing. Doing something we wouldn't usually do and trying something completely out of our comfort zone may be the exact thing that leads us to see just how loved and worthy we are. When we break the mold of fear, even in the most insignificant ways, we create new opportunities for healing.

TIME DOESN'T HEAL ALL WOUNDS

Coming face-to-face with the lies of our hearts is brutal. When we are waist-deep in the muck of the pain we've been avoiding for decades, we will do *anything* to find a way out.

For Kidist, the way out was through denial. Right before she came to the sober realization of how deeply her negative core belief was rooted in her life, she asked a question I hear all too often: "But this happened so long ago! Is it *really* a big deal?"

"Kidist, whether it happened yesterday or fifteen years ago, it's always a big deal if it shapes how you live."

She gave me a sarcastic smile, but I could tell I was getting through to her, so I continued.

"When you haven't eaten, do you get more or less hungry over time?" I asked her.

"Obviously more," she responded.

"So, what makes you believe that the things you needed as a child would become less painful and impactful over time?"

Silence.

"I never thought about it that way." She sighed.

"We never stop longing for what we need just because time passes. In fact, we'll feel the longing for those things more intensely."

Our souls continue to long for what we didn't receive. And the longer we go without it, the more it affects our spiritual health, just as prolonged hunger affects our physical health. Our needs don't disappear just because we refuse to acknowledge them. I shared this truth with Kidist, but it's a truth we all need to know. The need for safety, intimacy, peace, joy, companionship, and trust that you had when you were a baby, child, teen, and even adult will not go away until it's met. The hunger for love won't magically leave; you will just get hungrier and hungrier over time. The wounds that caused the lies you believe about yourself *did* happen long ago, but they are still relevant, they still matter, and yes, you still deserve to have them addressed.

In one session with Kidist, we discovered her negative core belief, after she'd spent months identifying and processing her destructive patterns of shrinking back, overgiving, and oversharing. Her relentless patterns of giving joyously in the moment only to feel exhausted and resentful later had drawn her to the edge, and she'd begun to experience compassion fatigue, emotional and physical exhaustion, leading to a diminished ability to empathize or feel compassion for others.

The more we dug into the ways she felt trapped in dysfunctional behaviors, the more we realized that what she thought was a heart of service was actually a posture of fear of rejection and low self-regard, which manifested in self-betrayal and enslavement to the people around her. For months we peeled back the layers of her fractured self that existed under the guise of service and humility. At church she won the Servant of the Year Award three years in a row. She led the setup and breakdown crews for all events and volunteered to help the children's ministry on her weekends off when they were short-staffed.

The more we met, the more Kidist realized that she did so much because she felt like she had to, not because she wanted to. There was a compulsive need to do because there was a lie playing like background music to her life—looping over and over. Playing for so long, she didn't even realize how loud it was.

If I were to randomly say to you, "Twinkle, twinkle little . . . ," before you could even take time to think, your brain would probably say *star*! Why? Because you've heard the song time and time again, and your brain has been wired to finish the song—even though you probably can't remember the first time you heard it. The same is true with our negative core beliefs. They are beliefs about who we are that we've heard so many times, rehearsed in so many ways, and felt so deeply that we probably say it or think it about ourselves without even realizing it.

To determine Kidist's negative core belief, I asked her to finish this sentence: "I am _____."

Immediately, she said "worthless." I brought to her awareness the reality that she was unable to rest because she could never access true silence or solitude. Quiet time was the environment where the songs of her unworthiness, failure, and shame played the loudest. She was stuck between being enslaved to the world around her and being deflated by the reality within her.

She wanted to change her external patterns because she thought it would change her life. But as long as the roots of her trauma, and the negative core beliefs it created, gripped the ground of her heart, the fruit of self-betrayal—incessant doing, resentment, and overgiving—would continue to grow.

What was Kidist to do with her negative core belief? Her "I am" statement? Well, she had to sit with it. Together we began to map out the places that validated that statement. I helped her connect her patterns to moments that made her feel like her negative core belief was true. I asked her about times when a favor was asked of her and she wanted to say no but couldn't. I asked her to share examples where she'd given to others when she didn't want to. I asked her to recall the emotions she felt. And I also asked her to think of the few times she did what *she* wanted. I asked her to remember times she felt proud or confident about how she cared for herself. Each question helped her see where her negative core belief played out in her life and also reminded her that the seeds of confidence, strength, clarity, and emotional honesty were there, even if she couldn't fully embody them the way she wanted to.

This is true of all of us. We all have our "I am" statements.

I am unlovable.
I am shameful.
I am unworthy.
I am destructive.
I am bad.

These statements are buried under years of dysfunctional behaviors and negative relational patterns. When we become unsatisfied with behaviors we can't stop and relational patterns we can't break, we have to look deeper. Though we can be tempted to believe we're just not disciplined enough, or don't have enough resources to change, the reality is, we feel compelled to engage in behaviors that burden and distress us because they reflect a deeper value we hold.

When we get to the core, we find that these lies have completely corroded our sense of self, our worthiness, and many times, our will to live. When we remember and revisit the original wound inflicted, we find a version of ourselves who doesn't believe that anything other than the lie can be true. A version of ourselves who looks nothing like the self we present to the world.

When our armor cracks and our protective patterns eventually fail us, our fractured self is exposed. Our insecurities and low self-esteem lay bare, no matter how confident we appear to the world.

We create a false self so that we can be loved, known, and respected, only to end up alone and afraid.

For some of us like Kidist, this cycle leads to overcommitting. We sign up for all volunteer opportunities, start new hobbies every month, lead teams at work, start small groups at church, and still feel like we're not doing enough. We fluctuate between being exhausted by our packed schedules and feeling like we don't do enough and need to fill our calendars more.

Though we're the ones who make our schedules, we feel suffocated by all the things we *need* to do and unsettled when there's nothing to do at all. In our actions the world sees strength and happiness, but internally a storm of chaos and turmoil rages.

I just want peace.
I need a break.
I just want to feel rested.

But when the opportunity for rest comes, the lies of our hearts—our negative core beliefs—get louder and louder. The screams of our unworthiness scare us into the action that drains us of our peace and denies our human need for acceptance based on who we are and not what we do. Though on the outside we are bold worshipers, who lead people into the promises of God effortlessly because we are full of faith for others, we are also shackled by despair regarding our own wounds. Both can be true. Both often are.

On the other hand, some of us respond to our negative core beliefs in a completely different way. Instead of running away from the lies about our identity, we become inwardly consumed with them. Instead of drowning out the song of unworthiness with our actions, with busyness, we're paralyzed by hopelessness, which leads us to draw inward and sing along to the voices of our angry and abusive parents, siblings, spouses, and friends. We've become accustomed to the sound of their criticism, because we've lived with them in our heads for so long. Suffocating under the emotional anguish that comes with being aware of just how wounded we've been, we draw inward.

If this is you, you may not share your true thoughts or opinions with others. Your outlets for pain are things no one is aware of—the three glasses of wine you need to fall asleep, the extra slices of pizza you mindlessly eat, or even the porn addiction you've never shared with anyone. Though many see a quiet and gentle person on the outside, you're spiritually exhausted and emotionally weary, resigned to the weight of your brokenness, with no will to live out loud.

HEALING FOR HOPELESSNESS

Whether we are always on the move or ever hidden away, at the core of our actions is terror, sadness, and even hopelessness—a hopelessness that comes from the lies that have fueled our lives without our permission. These lies affect every part of our lives, especially our relationship with God.

Healing means walking toward Jesus and slowly releasing our grip on the lies we feel are so true. We find a response in Jesus that is supernatural. One that pours out the glory of heaven on the version of ourselves that is tethered to the core lies we've carried from our trauma. The lies we believe about ourselves distort who we believe we're called to be. We wonder time and again, *Why can't I feel close to God?* The reality is, we can't feel close to anyone we're afraid of. It's a heartbreaking reality that we've been convinced out of our positions as coheirs with Christ.

When I first became a Christian, there was one Bible story that shook me to my core. In Matthew 7 Jesus preached a sermon to a crowd of people who had heard of His power and wisdom.

"Many will say to me on that day, 'Lord, Lord, did we not prophesy in your name and in your name drive out demons and in your name perform many miracles?' Then I will tell them plainly, 'I never knew you. Away from me, you evildoers!'" (vv. 22–23)

As a new believer who was preoccupied with doing the right things, this passage was like God had sent a message just for me, saying, *Hey! That performing thing you did before you knew Me? It doesn't work here. It means nothing at all. In fact, it won't get you any closer to Me, and it won't garner favor. It'll just draw you away from My love. Anything you don't do out of love is no good to Me. I want to be with you. Not just be served by you.*

I knew I was performing when I first read those words in the book of Matthew. I knew I was trying to earn God's love. I wanted to be the "good Christian," the serious one who was steeped in theology and knew the Greek and Hebrew translations of every word. God saw that I was more consumed with using His power to earn the love of others and less concerned with helping people see His tenderness as a reflection of His love for them.

Many of us bring our false selves into God's kingdom. We become obsessed with ordination, with titles like minister, pastor, elder, psalmist, and apostle. We are performing miracles, drawing the world to "ooh" and "ahh" at the anointing and maturity we have, all while forsaking the title of child. Yet it's Jesus who says if we don't receive His kingdom like a child, we won't receive it at all (Mark 10:15). We're often anxious and preoccupied with what we're doing wrong in our relationship with God instead of enjoying intimacy with Him. Few of us have a reference for anyone wanting to be near us just to be near us. It's hard to imagine that God would want to be with us "just because."

I'm convinced that God let the armor of my people-pleasing crack in order to remind me that the way I showed up in the world was not a reflection of who I actually was but rather a reflection of what I was so desperately protecting myself from: rejection and abandonment. He used the most common moments to help me see that no appearance of maturity would heal the reality of the childhood wounds I still carried. Time didn't heal my broken and fearful heart; I was just distanced from the reality of my pain by layers of defenses that made it easy to forget my heart was in dire condition. When I became aware of my heart's state, I thought the solution to the problem was to do what was done to me: shame it into correction, beat it into submission, and turn my back on it when it didn't change. It's amazing how we learn to hurt ourselves. Jesus is calling to the version of you that has been hiding in the dark. The weary and worn soul who has lived behind a shield of perfection and performance for too long. The person who has only gotten to see the light of day in moments of "success" tethered to anxiety.

Jesus longs for you to live in the light He's calling you into.

His call is a response to your silent cries, to the pleas for help that could come out only as tears, moans, and groans. He heard you. He *hears* you, and He did not forget. He still has good things for you. Not when you do more. Not when you get it together. He has it for you right now.

God knows that you only survived the cold of the world by covering yourself with coping mechanisms and dysfunctional behaviors. He knows you used them to protect yourself from the blizzard of fear and shame. You became codependent, forsaking your inner voice, becoming enslaved to others, and developing hyper-independence, because it was the only way you could adapt to the life you wanted to live in the midst of the lies you believed about yourself. You picked up patterns such as defining yourself by your emotions, as you found sadness and anger to be your only companions. You projected the pain of your past experiences onto others, so you could never feel blindsided by betrayal again. You returned to childhood emotional reactions that felt safe and didn't demand a heavy sense of responsibility. You intellectualized your way through life to avoid the pain your emotions led you into, and you displaced your rage onto people who were easier to lash out at than the people who actually hurt you.

After Kidist discovered her negative core belief, she realized just how many places it showed up in her life. She also became aware through our work of how many opportunities she had to show up for herself. Over time she came to understand that the experiences she had as a child didn't define her. Through our EMDR process she gained insight into the ways her past affected her, but she also gained insight into the moments of her life where she did feel a sense of worth and value. We challenged the lies of her past with the evidence of truth in the present, giving her a new perspective on herself and helping her develop new core beliefs.

We've learned to clothe ourselves with these defenses, like a winter jacket that we needed in a storm but are too afraid to take off when summer arrives. Seasons are changing. Winter is over! What once protected us is now suffocating us, stealing our ability to live freely. Though it feels like God is letting life strip us of safety when He unclothes us of our defenses, He's actually freeing us from the heavy burden we are trying to carry into a season of freedom. The things we've been wearing have protected us from hardship but have also kept us from knowing the wind on our skin and the warmth of the sun, the love of the Father. They've stolen our ability to know and experience what God has created us for, a reality God won't settle for even if we will.

What will we do with the frail person we find under all these patterns, pretenses, and illusions? Will we mock them? Scold them? Shame them? Or will we turn toward them, grabbing their feeble hand and telling them that we won't re-expose them to the abandonment they had to endure? Will we tell them to listen, mouthing the words that fall from heaven: "Come to me, all you who are weary and burdened, and I will give you rest" (Matthew 11:28)?

Will we listen to their pain rather than silence them? Will we empathize with their fear and tell them there's a safe place for it? Will we walk, shakily if we must, toward a Jesus whose eyes are filled with tears when we have none left? Will we lead them to gently lay their head on the chest of our Savior, who does not criticize who we've become but empathizes with how we arrived at such brokenness?

I hope, more than anything, that we will choose the latter.

Reflection Questions

1. Reflect on your own negative core beliefs.
2. Write down moments that made your negative core beliefs feel true.
3. Below I've created a basic checklist of possible negative core beliefs. Which ones cause a physical or emotional reaction? You may identify with several of these beliefs, or you may identify with none of them. Write them down, notice what emotions they bring up in you, and take time to journal about it.

Negative Core Belief Checklist

Survival
- ☐ I am going to die
- ☐ I am in danger
- ☐ I am overwhelmed

Shame (I am wrong)
- ☐ I don't deserve love
- ☐ I am a bad person
- ☐ I am terrible
- ☐ I am invisible
- ☐ I am worthless (inadequate)
- ☐ I am shameful
- ☐ I am not lovable
- ☐ I am not good enough
- ☐ I deserve only bad things
- ☐ I am permanently damaged
- ☐ I am ugly (my body is bad)
- ☐ I do not deserve good things
- ☐ I am stupid (not smart enough)
- ☐ I am insignificant (unimportant)
- ☐ I am a disappointment
- ☐ I deserve to die
- ☐ I deserve to be miserable
- ☐ I am different (don't belong)

Worth/Lovability
- ☐ I am unlovable
- ☐ I am worthless

- ☐ I am inadequate
- ☐ I am too difficult to love
- ☐ I am unwanted
- ☐ Nobody loves me
- ☐ Nobody wants me
- ☐ I am toxic
- ☐ I will always be rejected

Guilt (I've done something wrong)
- ☐ I've done something wrong (so everything wrong is my fault)
- ☐ I should have known better

Safety/Vulnerability
- ☐ I cannot be trusted
- ☐ I cannot trust myself
- ☐ I cannot trust my judgment
- ☐ I cannot trust anyone
- ☐ I cannot protect myself
- ☐ I am in danger
- ☐ It's not okay to feel (show) my emotions
- ☐ I cannot stand up for myself

Control/Choice
- ☐ I am not in control
- ☐ I am powerless (helpless)
- ☐ I am weak

- ☐ I am helpless
- ☐ I cannot get what I want
- ☐ I am a failure (will fail)
- ☐ I cannot succeed
- ☐ I am trapped in my life
- ☐ I have to be perfect (please everyone)
- ☐ I am inadequate
- ☐ I am ineffective
- ☐ I cannot trust anyone
- ☐ I can't change
- ☐ I am incapable
- ☐ I am vulnerable (unprotected)

Capability

- ☐ I am helpless
- ☐ I have no power
- ☐ I am weak
- ☐ I am insufficient on my own
- ☐ I cannot handle important things
- ☐ I am incompetent

Toxic/Shame

- ☐ I don't deserve to exist

part two

HEALING OUR WOUNDS

chapter six

DISCOVERING THE TRUTH: HOW DOES GOD RESPOND TO MY TRAUMA?

"Ooooh, you're in trouble . . ."

Growing up, anyone who heard those words knew the clock was ticking and impending wrath and punishment would soon come. I can't remember the last time I heard those actual words, but my body remembers the feeling of them—the racing heart, the desire to hide, and the stomach-clenching anxiety that intensified as the inevitable consequences drew near.

During my own personal therapy, I discovered I was living with the sense that I was always about to be in trouble with God. I'd left my faith out of so much of my healing process, because it was the context of so much of my trauma. There was too much to grieve. I felt like I couldn't bring it into the therapy room with me, so I often left it at the door.

Well, I tried to.

I found so much hope in the Jesus of the Bible, the Jesus who met me at rock bottom when I had no will to live. But when I became a Christian, the Jesus that was often taught to me was as mean as the people who had abused me. I believed He didn't care how I felt. I was a deep feeler and, man, was that demonized. Church was a place where I often felt shamed for feeling deeply. It was always a sign that something was wrong and never a reflection of how God made me. I can still hear the voices of the Bible study leaders and pastors telling me that God won't be pleased with me or bless me if I mess up or make a mistake. I told my therapist, "And I feel like my life is full of mistakes. I feel like I have to be perfect for Him to love me." Remembering the story of how I came to faith, she asked me to tell her again. As I shared in detail, I was reminded of the kindness of God.

"That sounds like a God of love and tenderness to me," she said.

He is.

The God I met in my lowest moment was One whose compassion and attention blew me away. But as I continued my faith journey through the lens of others and of my trauma, the kind Jesus, who made me want to live again, quickly morphed into a cold, demanding, and insensitive savior. This is who I began to see Jesus as—a man as mean as my bullies but with all the power in the world to save me. And since He *did* use it to save me, I had to see it as love, even when it felt just like the hate I'd known from others.

How can you lean on someone you think is annoyed with you? How can you trust someone you don't believe is safe—especially in your weakest moments? You can't, and you don't want to. Most of us wonder why our faith seems least powerful when we need it the most. In our despair, in our depression, in our sadness and hopelessness, the Jesus of our hearts is one of stone, not flesh and bone.

ROCK AND SAND

In Matthew 7 Jesus told a parable about a man who built his house on the rock and a man who built his house on sand. When the winds and waves crashed down on the house built on the rock, the house withstood the harsh weather. It stood amid the chaos, unshaken. When the storm raged around the house built on sand, it crumbled under the power of the storm. Jesus called the man who built his house on the rock wise, for listening and doing as Jesus directed. He called the man who heard His words and built his life on sand foolish.

When I think of this parable, I think of the identity I built in Christ based on my works. Time and time again Jesus made clear that it was His grace that saved me, His love that kept me. I knew His presence was meant to define me and the life I live. Still, through the lens of my trauma and negative core belief, I felt compelled to work in order to be loved. I *had* to earn it.

Brick by brick I built a new house, an identity designed to impress God instead of dwell with Him. It was about proving I could go the extra mile, showing Him how much more faithful I was than others. I didn't realize I was trying to earn what was already my birthright.

I brought the story and perspective of my trauma into my life with Christ. Same characters, same plot, different setting. Trauma tells us the things that are offered for free need to be worked for and convinces us to grow weary earning things that are meant to give us rest.

When I shared my feelings about God with my therapist, I began to realize my spiritual house, even in Christ, was still built on sand. The pain and heartbreak of the past had completely ravaged my identity. I had no clue who I was. The winds and waves had destroyed everything I knew of myself.

But at the bottom of my hope, once again, I was reintroduced to the same Jesus of tenderness. The Jesus of joy and hope. And He was asking me to build a house on the rock of who He is, not who I anticipated Him to be. He was offering me an opportunity to build a house with Him that would withstand even the fiercest storms. I wanted to, but I just couldn't figure out how I would. In the months and years to come, He would show me.

What's so interesting about the parable Jesus shared was that *both* builders heard Jesus. Both heard what He said, and yet both felt led to do different things. Both men heard Him, yet one was wise and one was foolish. I think the wise man was a man who *knew* Jesus. The foolish one was a man who just knew *about* Him.

My therapist asked me to close my eyes and recall the childhood moment that created my very first negative core belief—I am bad.

When I was around five, my family was at a party. My twin sister and I stood between two older women whom we called aunties but weren't actually my aunties. (If you're African, you already know.) One auntie asked, "Who is Panyin and who is Kakra?" (*Panyin* means "older twin" and *Kakra* means "younger twin" in Twi.)

"Kobe is Panyin," one woman said, "and Odua is Kakra."

"So who is the good twin, and who is the bad one?" the first woman asked. They both laughed intensely as if they knew something about us that we didn't.

"It's Kobe!" said one auntie. "Kobe is the bad one! She's always in trouble!"

I remember feeling sad and sick as my stomach dropped. I wanted to say something to protest, but in my culture, you don't talk back to elders.

I don't even think I realized how much I internalized that moment until I was in my twenties. I'd lived a life through the lens of being bad. Every mistake I made and every moment I disappointed my parents was evidence of what felt like the truth: I am bad. It was the story I lived in; I was the villain. But when I met Jesus, I began to hope that I could be more than that. But that hope quickly slipped away.

Back in my therapist's office, I brought the image to my mind as I had for many months. The room. My sister. My aunties. The laughing. The pain.

"I want you to imagine that Jesus is in the room with you," my therapist said. "Where is He in this scene?"

"He's standing in the corner of the party." Although I knew I was in the therapy room, the image I saw as my eyes were closed was so vivid.

"And what is He doing?" she asked.

"He's looking at me. He seems sad, but now He's walking over," I told her. I began to weep. She stayed silent, knowing something powerful was happening.

"He held my hand and pulled me away from the two women," I said through tears. "He interrupted the auntie before she could call me bad, and He kneeled down and told me that He sees me as good."

WHEN JESUS IS IN THE ROOM

This experiential exercise my therapist walked me through was a paradigm shift. At the core of the exercise was something she was ushering me into that was greater than recalling my past to find the bright side of my pain. She was helping me invite God into the healing of one of the most formative moments of my life, by helping me access emotions and negative core beliefs attached to that moment while I also focused on what I knew of the character of Jesus. She invited me to see Jesus as a participant of my painful memory by asking me to imagine Him in it. Through that imagination, I gained access to the spiritual reality that He *was* there, and He had something to show me.

This is one of several ways we can invite Jesus into our traumatic experiences, giving Him opportunity to do what only He can do. That presence, that experience, that intangible tenderness that wrapped my soul in peace and flooded it with acceptance gave me the wisdom I needed to build my house on the rock of Jesus' words. This presence banished the image of Jesus that was used to scare and oppress me, back into the darkness where it belonged. It opened my eyes to the true presence of my Savior, who is deeply attuned to my pain and longing to restore my broken heart. It was everything I'd longed for and nothing I expected.

So much of my walk with God was marked by fear. Stained with the idea that if I didn't start getting it right (whatever "it" is), God would punish me, abandon me, and rescind every prophecy and promise over my life. My destructive patterns, fueled by my traumas and negative core beliefs, made it hard for change to happen. When I was "good," I felt on top of the world. But the smallest mistake made me question whether God still loved me. I didn't know how God felt about my trauma. Was He annoyed? Did He not care? Was He as insensitive as the people I'd encountered? In that session with my therapist, I got to discover something more powerful than my perfection.

To the greatest terrors and traumas of our lives, God offers us the one thing we long for the most, the one thing the world often withholds: tenderness. My experience with my therapist didn't only change my spiritual perspective of God. That encounter with Jesus also affected the biological chaos I'd experienced in my body for so long due to my trauma. I felt peace in my body, too, not just in my spirit.

To the greatest terrors and traumas of our lives, God offers us the one thing we long for the most, the one thing the world often withholds: tenderness.

TENDERNESS

Songwriter Marvin Sapp wrote,

> *He saw the best in me*
> *When everyone else around*
> *Could only see the worst in me*

Those words never felt truer to me.

Jesus gave me acceptance when I expected rejection, and tenderness when I expected judgment. His actions expanded my understanding of how I could be valued when I felt sad, inadequate, and alone. The moment I realized Jesus was in the room initiated the rewiring of my brain's expectations of how God sees me. It created new neurological pathways of possibilities of what I could expect when I was struggling to change or when I felt overwhelmed with the pain of the past. He revealed the option of being motivated by love rather than punishment, by acceptance rather than fear of rejection. We learn to think poorly of ourselves through repetition; we learn how loved we are by God through repetition too. One moment can change everything. But often it doesn't; it's the many small moments of acceptance from God that rival the years of self-hatred and fear.

We need moment after moment of God's tenderness. That's what drowns out the fear. That's what shows us there's a greater motivator for change than hating ourselves. No change motivated by fear lasts. If it does, it's always at the expense of our peace.

If you've ever wondered how God responds to your trauma, here is your answer: God responds to your neurological, emotional, relational, and spiritual reality of terror with tenderness, compassion, and provision. He's not only concerned with your spiritual standing but with your biological existence. He wants you to know peace in your body. He opens us to the biological capacity for it by giving us experiences that refute the fears of our souls. He's attuned to the anxiety and aware of the depression that keeps coming back. He knows what you feel, because He created the systems that allow you to feel. He lived a life that utilized these systems too.

In Numbers 11, Moses was leading the people of God through the desert. Overwhelmed by the task of leading and tending to the Israelites, Moses shared his frustration and desperation with God, saying, "I cannot carry all these people by myself; the burden is too heavy for me. If this is how you are going to treat me, please go ahead and kill me" (vv. 14–15).

In his utter desperation, Moses, a hero of the faith, expressed what we call *suicidal ideation*, thinking about dying. Most of us come from faith traditions that would respond to someone, especially a leader, who expresses suicidal ideation with theological perspectives about whether suicidal ideations are sin or not. Whether that person is going to hell or not. Whether that person is fit to lead or not. But God did something completely different.

He didn't even address the suicidal ideation. He didn't rebuke Moses for expressing such candid anger. God's first response was this: "Bring me seventy of Israel's elders who are known to you as leaders and officials among the people. Have them come to the tent of meeting, that they may stand there with you" (v. 16). God responded to the cause of the stress, not the symptom that arises because of it. God's heart toward those who are at the end of their rope and completely overwhelmed is not judgment or punishment. It's tenderness. It's provision. It's an open ear, heart, and hand.

God's response to Moses isn't a one-time thing. We see His heart toward those who are emotionally wounded, exhausted, and depleted in His interaction with Elijah in 1 Kings. As Elijah fled from those who wanted to kill him, he came to a place where he was desperate and weary, saying, "'Take my life; I am no better than my ancestors.' Then he lay down under the bush and fell asleep" (19:4–5). Here we see suicidal ideation again.

When Elijah decided to sleep, God didn't send him an angel to tell him to get up and pray. God sent an angel to enhance his rest, to fill his belly, and to usher him into better sleep. What a concept.

The angel then said, "'Get up and eat, for the journey is too much for you'" (v. 7). When I first read the words "the journey is too much for you," I didn't understand why it was there. *Of course the journey is too much for him!* I thought. *He already said that.*

The angel used a skill called *reflective listening*—a therapeutic tool used by therapists to connect to clients. It lets the clients know that we hear the words they are saying, we understand the emotions behind them, and we connect to their experiences. The angel said back to Elijah the very words he used to express his feelings. The angel didn't do this to inform Elijah; he said it to let him know that God heard his cries. God was listening.

God understood that the emotional distress was connected to a physical need.

God met the needs of Moses and Elijah. He didn't dismiss their feelings as silly, dumb, or a lack of faith.

It was as if the angel were saying to Elijah, "I see what you're feeling, and it matters to God. I see that you're dysregulated; I see that you're overwhelmed. I'm going to do something about it. I am going to give you rest. I am going to lighten your burden. I am going to show you tenderness in the midst of your despair instead of shaming you for experiencing it." Again, God did not respond to the suicidal ideation, but He did address the cause of it by lightening the load, giving rest, and assuring safety.

When Jesus said, "Come to me, all you who are weary and burdened, and I will give you rest" (Matthew 11:28), He meant it. The rest for our souls is not figurative, flowery language. It's an actual reality He gives. He interrupts the narratives that make us feel like life isn't worth living and offers us refuge.

When we are in despair, God provides. When we are depressed, God offers tenderness. Once Elijah experienced the tenderness of God in his darkest moment, he was strengthened to keep going. And Moses, with the support of the elders, continued to lead. The weight of our trauma doesn't disqualify us from what God calls us to, but it can impair our ability to show up the way we need to. When we share our pain with God, he provides for the journey. He cares for our souls.

WHAT DO YOU BELIEVE ABOUT GOD?

I think many of us don't believe in the tenderness of God because we haven't experienced it yet. In our brokenness, we know we have done things we're not proud of, and rather than finding refuge in Jesus, all we see is judgment.

Who we believe God to be can positively or negatively affect our mental and emotional health. When we don't get to experience Him, we are more likely to echo the narratives of our pain instead of the truth of His loving care. Below is a quick activity you can utilize to process some of the deeply held beliefs you have about how God responds to you in your experience of trauma. In the previous chapter, we went through an activity that helped us acknowledge some negative emotions that need to be addressed (pp. 92–93). Feel free to reference those emotions in this activity:

When I feel _____,
I expect God to respond to me with _____,
Which causes me to want to respond
    by _____.

The tenderness you're imagining God giving you is real. It's already being offered. It's being extended to you, right now as you read this. Though you may feel like you're imagining it, you're only becoming awakened to it. Let that tenderness and love touch every wound like salve for your soul.

When our identities are shaken and topple over under the storm of trauma, it can seem like the end, but in our grief God pulls us deeper into the very things our souls thirst for. When we open our hearts to grieve with Jesus, we get to experience the divine comfort that He creates specifically for our deep wounds. That tenderness opens the door to the restoration and transformation of our identities after they've been battered by the pain of the past. Out of love and acceptance, we can step into new patterns of living.

The LORD is my shepherd; I shall not want.

He makes me lie down in green pastures.

He leads me beside still waters.

He restores my soul.

He leads me in paths of righteousness

for his name's sake.

Even though I walk through the valley of the shadow

of death,

I will fear no evil,

for you are with me;

your rod and your staff,

they comfort me. (Psalm 23:1–4 ESV)

HE MAKES ME LIE DOWN IN GREEN PASTURES

God allows us to become fully awakened to the weight of the pain we're carrying. And instead of asking more *of* us, He gives more *to* us, by inviting us to rest with Him with all the burdens we carry. He speaks to the lie that we can receive kindness and tenderness only after we've become good enough.

God restores us by establishing His role in this process of healing. He will lead us. We lack nothing, because He will provide it all. In a world where we're told to pull ourselves up by the bootstraps as we take full responsibility for the brokenness we experienced, His message of tenderness restores the original image that trauma inverted. It takes the burden of healing and restoration off our shoulders and out from under our feet.

We get to be sheep. Sheep don't have to worry about anything but being sheep. The shepherd tells them where to go. He points to the food; he leads them to water. He tells them to stop; he tells them to go. You don't have to conjure up Jesus' tenderness toward you. He'll bring you to it, show you how to rest in it, and teach you how to drink of it.

God restores us by establishing His role in this process of healing.

HE LEADS ME BESIDE STILL WATERS

God lets us wade in His presence as we are surrounded by the beauty of His love. His tenderness recalibrates our emotional discernment by helping us see that, though there may be a monster in the room, there's also a Savior who offers us an embrace to rest in.

As He leads us away from the doing and distracting, we get to simply exist as beloved. He leads us beside peace. He stays with us; He guides us beside still waters as we see reflections of ourselves and Him in them. This stillness with Jesus breaks every illusion we've held as truth. It shatters every idea that dampens His glory.

Healing is not always in the doing. It's not in the striving. Healing won't come from trying harder; it won't come from engaging in the same behaviors that made us feel useless and discarded.

Instead, healing will come from leaning in to God—from dwelling with Him, without empty flattery or religious routine. We lean in by opening our hearts to what God wants to offer us in our hardship, rather than what we can do to please Him in it. Healing comes through dwelling with Him in silence, or simply repeating a breath prayer in our anxiety as we, in our weariness, leave the work of the heart to the Holy Spirit. That dwelling allows for the cries of our hearts that have been buried under brokenness.

If you're wondering what it looks like practically to lean in, there are multiple spiritual disciplines that can help us experience the tenderness of God wherever we are. Some of my personal favorites are centering prayer, breath prayer, examen, and lament. We'll talk about and use some of these later on in the book, but all of these can be accessed in *Spiritual Disciplines Handbook* by Adele Ahlberg Calhoun. This book is an incredible resource for people who want to investigate even more ways to intimately connect with God.

Knowing that God wanted to meet my sadness and shame with tenderness and provision left me hungry to see more of where He was in my story. I found myself journaling and praying over moments where my heart was broken. I'd close my eyes, envisioning myself experiencing the emotions I struggled to move through, and would then ask God, "Show me how You're responding to me right now." I'd often get an image of a caramel-skinned Jesus holding my hand, hugging me as I wept, or weeping with me.

On those hard days I utilize *centering prayer*—a contemplative prayer that allows me to quiet scattered and anxious thoughts in the center of God's presence. Through intentional, deep diaphragmatic breathing, I center myself in the presence of God. I choose a word that best described what my heart needs to hear and receive from God. "Safe" is often my word. As I breathe, I speak that word to myself, over and over, to every present thought that surfaces, every feeling of being unsafe. I meet every anxious thought with the truth of my standing in Christ. I am safe in Him.

I often lie with my head on a pillow as I envision myself reclined on the chest of Jesus. I imagine what His tunic feels like, as I visualize my head rising and falling with the rhythm of His breath, my heartbeat in sync with His. The imagery decreases my pulse, opens my heart, and gives me access to the tender presence of Jesus.

HE RESTORES MY SOUL

God restores with gentleness. Exodus 34:6 recounts the first time God described His character to the people of Israel. Moses proclaimed to all the people of Israel that God was "the LORD, the LORD, the compassionate and gracious God, slow to anger, abounding in love and faithfulness."

Sit with that for a minute. "Compassionate" is the first word God ever used to describe Himself. The word *compassionate* in Hebrew is *rakhum* (v.) or *rakhamim* (n.), a term that derives from the Hebrew word for womb (*rehem*). The word *compassion* in the Jewish world is centered in someone's core, giving us the imagery of God's attentiveness to us as a reflection of a mother's deep attunement and love for her child.

The word also translates to being "deeply moved." Our cries of despair are like strong kicks and movements in the womb of God. The word *rakhum* refers to feelings, but more specific, feelings that move someone to action. It is the word used most to describe God's actions, motivated by His emotions.

When the Israelites were oppressed in Egypt, God heard their cries and was motivated by His compassion, His *rakhamim*, to rescue them.[1] In a similar way, God is attuned to your cries. They are movements in His womb, kicks so strong He gets up and does something about it.

The word *compassion* directly translates to the phrase "suffer with." Whenever Jesus shows compassion, He enters *into* our suffering with us. He draws us out of cycles of destruction by meeting us in them, even when we want to stay. He doesn't let us settle for simply surviving. He invites us into His love and awakens our desires as a response to our unspoken prayers. He suffers *with* us; He's moved by our cries, and He desires to hear them. When He does hear them, He won't turn away.

When you feel like you can't come into God's presence today because you made a mistake yesterday, know that your mistakes are ever sinking in a sea of forgiveness. They are searching for a bottom they'll never find. When you think God is mad at you because you didn't read the Bible long enough or pray hard enough in your quiet time, know that every morning, waves of grace and mercy crash at your feet. Before you do a thing, He offers you an unending grace that draws you into the current of love that leads to intimacy. For every lie that reappears in moments of being triggered and overwhelmed, know that God never gets tired of whispering the truth to your soul.

If you're too depressed to pray, the Holy Spirit intercedes on your behalf with wordless groans. If you're too sad to worship, the heavenly hosts are surrounding you with a song of deliverance.

God doesn't want more from you. He's giving more to you.

EVEN THOUGH I WALK THROUGH THE VALLEY

Following Jesus rarely means you get to avoid the valleys of your trauma, but He prepares you with His loving tenderness to trust that the paths He leads you down are the right ones, even when they lead back to the valleys you so desperately wanted to escape. The tenderness of a God who lays us down in lush, green pastures, and the compassion of a God who leads us beside still waters to restore our souls, allows us to reflect the sentiments of David when he courageously said, "I will fear no evil."

Many of us won't believe in the protection of God until we know the tenderness of God. Trauma can create in us a cold and callous demeanor that mirrors the very essence of the people who wounded us. It's interesting how, when we don't let our wounds heal properly, we become what we are so preoccupied with protecting ourselves from. We become selfish, and because we were left unprotected by others for so long, we become unconcerned with protecting others. We become preoccupied with our needs because our needs weren't met by others. As a result, we forget how to show up for others.

Our trauma can lead us to miss the mark God has for us. But for me, every path of correction God has set me on has been lit with a compassion that shook my very being. Every moment God asked me to let go of my bitterness, He did so by reminding me that He knew my pain and wanted freedom for me.

YOUR ROD AND YOUR STAFF COMFORT ME

In the ancient world, a shepherd's staff was used to rescue sheep when they were in distressing situations. It was meant to guide them when they went astray. The rod was used to protect the sheep from predators, defending them from harm. It was also used to count the sheep. To keep track of everyone. To keep an eye on every member of the flock.

Though trauma has made you believe that God uses His power to harm you, He's actually using His power to save you, to keep you close. He's not beating you with a rod of discipline when you're wounded and vulnerable, like so many of us have been taught. He's defending you from harm and keeping His loving eye on you. This is what we can find our comfort in, as David mentioned earlier.

And this is what I got to experience in my therapy session. A God who shows up. A God who pulls me away. A God who doesn't delight in my pain.

Many of us cannot hold or touch the things that most wounded our souls. They were intangible—things like words, postures, and tones that communicated things that cut us deeply. But we *can* remedy the wounds of our identity. Presence restores rejection. Presence restores betrayal. Presence restores abandonment.

YOU ARE WITH ME

My toddler was having a rough day. After being told it was time to go to bed, he grabbed his favorite toy and threw it at the wall as hard as he could. The roomful of relatives froze. They preemptively braced and winced, expecting me to spank him or scream at him.

Instead, I got down on one knee, took a deep breath, and said, "You're having a hard time, aren't you? You must have some really big emotions in your body."

He nodded, then hugged me and put his head on my shoulder. "Mommy," he said, "I'm tired."

I already knew. After many months of screaming, demanding, and popping him on the hand for expressing himself in ways we saw as unacceptable, I saw something brewing beneath the surface of his actions. He would say things like "I'm bad." It broke my heart that our responses to him encouraged that self-perspective. I knew from experience what it was like to go through life feeling that way about yourself, so we made a change. The more tender we are with our son in his distress and frustration, the more courageous and assured he is of himself. He feels safe with us. His personality shines, and every day he gets to show up as himself, without fear.

I have been able to experience this courage in my own relationship with God. There's something about the tenderness of His presence that strengthens us, fortifies us, and gives us access to courage we thought we'd never possess. There's something about feeling safe with someone—about feeling safe with Jesus—that makes you feel like you can do things you once felt were impossible.

A HARD AND BEAUTIFUL TRUTH

I desperately want to be able to tell you that God always keeps you beside still waters. I want to say that He restores your soul in those places alone, but the greater story of redemption takes us through dark valleys, so we can reclaim and redeem what was lost and what was wounded. When we realize just how far into darkness the love and power of Jesus reach, we become assured, again and again, that there is nothing in the world that will separate us from His love. As we revisit the emotional realities that were created by the things that wounded us, we'll discover a patience like nothing we've ever experienced.

In His tenderness, God ushers us home. He restores the God-breathed, infinitely unique spirit He created within us. Just as a parent's words shape a child, God reshapes us, giving us a corrective emotional experience in Him. We get to reexperience intimacy as safe rather than terrifying. We receive honor for our childlikeness, rather than shame; we receive love instead of rejection and abandonment. He corrects the wounds of our souls with His love. He provides the unyielding rock of His tenderness as the foundation for the new lives made of new perspectives and new patterns we are building with Him. He blesses us with things we've long dreamed of but never imagined we'd receive.

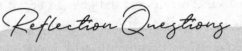

Reflection Questions

1. What are some of the deeply held beliefs you have about how God responds to you in your trauma?
2. How do you imagine God would respond to you in your trauma and pain if you imagined Him in the room with you?
3. What would God's tenderness give you courage to embrace or let go of in your life?
4. Utilize centering prayer or the meditative prompt of laying your head on Jesus' chest. Do this practice for two minutes. Journal about what you notice physically, emotionally, and spiritually. Remember, these are all practices. They may not feel helpful or natural the first time you try them. Still, continue to utilize them if you feel led to.

chapter seven

RECOGNIZING TRIGGERS:
WHY DO I REACT THIS WAY?

"I'm so tired of living this way."

Tola (Toh-lah) was a quiet, gentle woman who loved the arts, music, and film. She was universally liked by the people around her, but felt deeply unknown. People often applauded her for her faithfulness to church, her amicable posture, and her accommodating demeanor. She was always invited out to events by friends and leaders in the community and was highly regarded by everyone. Tola loved being respected by her family, friends, and community. She loved being spoken well of by them. But when she was alone, she was overwhelmed with loneliness.

Tola rarely spoke up when she was treated poorly and never enforced her boundaries. She always went with the flow, for the sake of keeping the peace around her—at the expense of the peace within her. In one session, Tola and I spoke about an upcoming trip she had planned with her family. "I really don't want to go on this trip." She sighed.

"You dread it," I reflected back to her.

"Yes!" she exclaimed. "Every time I travel with my family it feels like my job is to make everyone feel good, especially my dad."

Tola lived the life of a people pleaser. She desperately wanted to break out of the mold of doing whatever people asked of her but was terrified of the rejection and harsh words she might face if she stood up. She loved how highly she was spoken of but hated the price she had to pay for it.

She loved making other people happy, but it drained her, and she struggled to develop a clear perspective of what she wanted in life amid the voices of the people she wanted to please. As she grew exhausted by the role of perfection she played in others' lives, Tola struggled more and more with intense anxiety, which led her into a cycle of withdrawing from her friends and faith community for months at a time.

During our time together, she began to realize how terrified she was of having to endure other people's disappointment. "Okay," I said. "I want you to take a second to close your eyes and notice what you're experiencing in your body as you think about the dread you feel regarding this trip." I let her breathe through her developing awareness. "Now I want you to think back to a moment in the last few weeks when you felt these same bodily sensations."

A tear formed, then rolled down her cheek. She took a deep breath, then opened her eyes. "I thought about my childhood," she whispered. "I saw how my parents screamed at and spoke about my siblings whenever they shared their thoughts and opinions. They never put their hands on us, but I was terrified of being on the receiving end of their wrath." During a previous session, Tola had shared with me that she had an okay relationship with her father. Though she loved him deeply, she was deathly afraid of disappointing him.

At a young age, she discovered that if she did everything he wanted and even anticipated what he wanted, his anger would subside. Then, he was a fun and pleasant person to be around.

Tola was convinced that her childhood was completely normal and that she didn't have any trauma from it. She only saw abuse through the lens of being physically or sexually harmed. And since she hadn't experienced that, she struggled to see the relational patterns she adopted from childhood as traumatic at all. In the past, when I'd gently led her to see how the terror she felt as a little girl still shows up in her life today, she'd been hesitant and resistant. Today, she was ready.

"Every time I talk to him, I'm always on edge. It feels like my life revolves around his anger. Somehow, I became the person who was responsible for making sure he didn't blow up on everyone else in the family. Now everyone else in the family makes me the peacekeeper."

"What emotions does that bring up for you?"

Her eyes shifted to my handy laminated emotions wheel. She grabbed it and ran her fingers over each word until she stopped.

"Wow. Well, first of all, I think I feel rage on a daily basis." I nodded as she continued to search for her original answer. "He makes me feel abandoned and dismissed," she said. "Being around my dad makes me feel like my life and desires don't matter apart from what they offer him. Like who I am doesn't matter at all, only what I do."

"I'm hearing you say that you feel trapped in cycles of hiding your true desires in order to please the people around you. When you feel overwhelmed from serving everyone else, without being able to freely be yourself, you experience depressive symptoms and isolate. It seems like you're seeing that this is a cycle that started in your childhood..."

She rubbed her hands together and hung her head, sniffling back tears.

"Tola," I leaned in. "I'm also hearing that among all the people who like you, there are few you feel know you, which makes you feel like your life doesn't matter."

Her cry became audible. "Sometimes I just want to disappear!" she blurted through tears. "I don't want to kill myself, but sometimes living just seems like too much. I feel like I'm suffocating. I'm just tired."

Many of us think the key indicator that leads a person to consider suicide is sadness. I've noticed that it's often overwhelming exhaustion. Tola and I discussed the difference between wanting to die—suicidal ideation—and actually planning to go through with the action—suicidal intent. She shared that she had experienced only ideation. We created a safety plan, engaged in hope-developing interventions, and made space for her to share her thoughts without shame.

In the following months, I walked with Tola through understanding her triggers, and we began the journey of processing her childhood trauma. She came to understand that as a child she had internalized her father's leaving as a fault of her own. She knew she deserved to live a life that reflected her values; she just didn't know how to actually act on that knowledge. Tola came to see that she still carried the childhood perspective that controlling her father's outbursts was her responsibility. Even when she tried to do everything perfectly, he would still blow up, causing her to feel intense fear and guilt for not controlling the situation. The guilt of not controlling his mood ate at her, throwing her into patterns of people-pleasing, to make sure everyone around her was happy even if she wasn't. But like clockwork, being enslaved to the thoughts and feelings of the people around her exhausted her, causing her to withdraw and isolate.

Even when her father was in a good mood, Tola was triggered

by his presence. His joy made her feel anxious about what might set him off. His anger ignited feelings of guilt, shame, and absolute fear, as he berated her and her family when things didn't go his way.

She didn't want to go on this trip, because she knew she would be triggered.

TRIGGERED

The word *trigger* has, without a doubt, become a buzzword, as our culture seeks to gain a deeper understanding of mental health and trauma. Unfortunately, everything that becomes quickly and widely understood is usually oversimplified.

When I hear people talk about their triggers, they mention moments that make them feel angry, or uncomfortable. However, triggers are much more complex than simply experiencing what many of us label as negative emotions. The literal definition of a trigger is "a stimulus that elicits a reaction."[1] Triggers are biological and relational reminders that something painful and confusing happened to us or around us in a way that affects our present experiences. They are evidence that our bodies store memories of the pain we've endured, even when those painful moments are long gone.

Sometimes we only think of triggers as the loud fireworks that make a combat veteran slam to the ground, but triggers are that and so much more. They are complex, nuanced, and incredibly personal. Triggers are any stimuli that elicit a reaction related to a past negative experience. They can be sounds, smells, colors, textures, sights, and tastes. They can be words, phrases, songs, physical motions, flavors, and images. Though they vary, they all create the same product—they bring you back into the painful moments of the past.

Triggers are not just about remembering past pain; they are about reexperiencing past pain as if it were happening in the present. We may sweat, cry, scream, jump, or experience an endless combination of reactions to things that have happened in the past but are being experienced in the present.

Let's say you have been taught all your life that you are safe with your mother and father. But one day while riding with your mom and dad, you get into a horrific accident that injures all of you severely, leaving you hospitalized for weeks. Before the accident, the world you lived in was built on the principle that as long as you were with your parents, you were safe. The moment your car collided with another, wounding you and the people you believed you were safe with, your brain and body began silently processing how you could be so severely wounded with your parents in the car.

As a child, you may not be able to make sense of this seemingly simple idea. And since your whole world is built on the idea that you are safe with your parents, seeing your parents severely wounded may not just harm your body but set your mind into a panic, as every idea of safety is put into question by the accident.

As years pass, you hate to drive your car. Beyond that, you trust no one and begin to anticipate danger everywhere. Unaware of the effects of the accident, you don't realize that you lost the ability to trust anyone with your safety after that event. This leads to being triggered by lack of control into states of rage, panic, and terror—all sensations that haven't been cognitively connected to the accident, but which originated there. These feelings are stored in your body. The lack of control that came from the car accident now becomes the bullhorn that calls forth all the unresolved emotions that still exist but haven't been fully processed.

Triggers are biological and relational reminders that something painful and confusing happened to us or around us in a way that affects our present experiences.

Tola's life was built on the idea that if she just did everything perfectly, she could prevent her father's angry outbursts. Because, as a child, she could not make sense of the fact that the person who was meant to keep her safe was also the person who terrified her, she oversimplified the solution to the problem: *I'll make sure that I make him happy, so he'll stop being upset.* Her childhood experience left her with unresolved feelings of sadness, anger, and confusion, which were suppressed when she made people feel good, but which were drawn back to the surface of her life when she experienced dread and exhaustion from realizing that no amount of perfection could control someone else's emotions.

One might think Tola would be triggered only if she remembered a specific moment, but triggers are much more sophisticated than that. When we have traumatic experiences, our brains and bodies memorize the contexts in which we experienced that pain, to anticipate when it may happen again so we can protect ourselves. Triggers validate our negative core beliefs and shock us back into the biological environment of our deepest wounds. There are no skills that can make a person stop themselves from ever being triggered again. But there are skills that allow us to cope with the triggers until we are less and less disarmed by them and desensitized to the previously painful memories they bring us.

THE BIOLOGY OF TRIGGERS

If we really want to understand triggers, we have to first look at how the human nervous system is set up. Our nervous system is separated into two smaller systems: the central nervous system (which includes our brain and spinal cord) and the peripheral nervous system (which consists of the somatic nervous system and the autonomic nervous system). The somatic nervous system is involved in the voluntary movement of our skeletal muscles, while the autonomic includes involuntary functions, such as our nerves, which regulate the automatic functions in our bodies that help us stay alive and healthy (like breathing and keeping your heart going).

The autonomic nervous system is important as we gain a deeper understanding of triggers. This system is split up into two different systems: the sympathetic nervous system (SNS) and the parasympathetic nervous system (PNS).[2] The SNS is activated in our bodies in the face of great physical exertion, threat, or perceived threat. This includes moments like lifting weights, running, and sexual activity, but it also kicks in during incredibly stressful moments, like running from danger, fighting off an attacker, or facing an abuser. The PNS is activated in times of recovery and rest. This includes moments like prayer, relaxation, meditation, sleep, or spending time with your loved one.

Ideally these two systems are meant to complement each other, collaborating to ensure our survival. No one system is meant to dominate. Without the SNS there would be no excitement or response to danger and without the PNS there would be no rest, and our hearts would give out from overexertion. Together they create the perfect survival system, which allows us to enjoy life and connect to others while having the tools to protect ourselves from danger.

When our SNS is activated, it prepares our bodies to protect against threat and danger. This response manifests in either fight or flight or freeze. In the first two responses, your muscles tense, your heart rate increases, your sensitivity to pain decreases, your pupils dilate, you become hyperaware of your surroundings, and you may feel shaky and clammy as stress hormones flood your body and as blood is rushed to your head, heart, and extremities to prepare for action. Here's how the fight and flight responses differ:

Fight

The *fight* response is the adaptive automatic trauma response that occurs when we engage a perceived threat around us. When we face perceived threats, we respond with aggression signaled by the following:

- tight jaw or grinding of the teeth
- urge to hit or harm someone or something
- feeling intense anger
- yelling and screaming
- crying
- glaring at people or conversing angrily
- attacking or confronting the source of the danger

Flight

The *flight* response is the adaptive automatic trauma response that occurs when we try to escape the perceived threat before us. When we are confronted with perceived threats, we escape from danger by distancing ourselves in these ways:

- physically avoiding a person, place, or thing

- distracting ourselves from the issue at hand
- constantly moving legs, feet, and arms
- exiting places when we feel overwhelmed

Freeze

The *freeze* response is the adaptive automatic trauma response that occurs when we become immobilized by fear when facing a threat. Though the parasympathetic system is often attributed with rest and relaxation, when fighting or fleeing potential danger is not an option, our body can go into the freeze response. This utilizes the parasympathetic system to decrease the body's heart rate and release hormones that decrease pain sensitivity, so the person is experiencing a form of physical or emotional paralysis, unable to move or act.

In the freeze response, our fear displays itself in the following ways:

- inability to move
- pale skin
- loss of sense of time
- inability to speak
- feeling stiff, heavy, cold, or numb
- loud, pounding heart
- decreasing of heart rate
- feeling trapped in your body

These trauma responses happen on their own, without our control or permission. Think of the last time you were surprised. Maybe you tripped over something you didn't see or were shocked by the need to brake suddenly while driving. At that moment, all the body responses leapt into action without your even thinking about it.

This is the biological reality of being triggered. It's having our mind and body fully convinced of life-threatening danger in a way that prepares the body to leap into action or freeze in fear, even if we're not aware of what we're defending ourselves from. This is a powerful and beautiful biological response, which God created to keep us safe from danger. But when we have trauma, our responses go haywire. Our body perceives immediate danger where there is none and shocks us out of a state of rest by activating our trauma responses at the drop of a dime.

What makes triggers so harmful to us? They prolong and misattribute states of panic and terror that were made only for very specific moments and make them an everyday occurrence. Triggers disorient us; they make us feel like we're on fire when there is no flame. When we are living in the present, our bodies are utilizing our PNS, the rest and digest system. This is the biological state we are supposed to be most acquainted with. Sadly, many of us aren't. The PNS directs blood to our core and digestive systems, activates our immune system, decreases our heart rate, and slows the intense contractions of our lungs. This is the biological system at work when we are laughing with friends, taking a nap, watching our favorite show, or reading a book. When we are living in a safe reality, our bodies are in peaceful homeostasis.

But what happens when we are constantly reminded of our trauma or always feel under attack? Well, the SNS stays on, overexposing us to adrenaline, cortisol, and other stress hormones. This type of overexposure prevents the body's ability to rest and engage in daily functions.

When we have unresolved wounds that we haven't integrated into our lives, the constant fear that disintegration creates in our bodies creates a miscommunication between our brain and the systems that set off our sympathetic responses. This causes them to activate in times when they shouldn't, which results in our bodies functioning in our trauma responses too often and for too long. Health problems result, including the following:

- anxiety
- depression
- digestive problems
- headaches
- muscle tension and pain
- heart disease, heart attack, high blood pressure, and stroke
- sleep issues
- weight gain
- memory and concentration impairment

It is important to understand the biology of being triggered because there are so many myths about triggers, especially in communities of faith. Not every undesirable response is a trigger, but the uneducated can be impatient, annoyed, and frustrated when people express being legitimately triggered. I've seen leaders and ministers tell people to "get over it" and "just stop being triggered," as if the automatic biological responses to pain are somehow a reflection of their faithfulness, morality, obedience, or trust in God. Statements like this eclipse the compassion and tenderness of Jesus, making it hard to come to Him, especially when we're told that those heaping burdens on us are representatives of the God who created us.

Here's the truth: God is not angry at you for being triggered. He empathizes with you, responds to you with compassion, and sends His Comforter to be with you in times of uncontrollable anger and despair. When we don't understand what triggers are, we don't understand how to connect to people who experience them. We don't know how to connect to ourselves because, at some point in time, we all experience triggers. And when we deny mercy to others, it's often because we've first denied it to ourselves.

God created these biological systems. God knows the deep intricacies of them. And God is much wiser than those who oversimplify the pain and terror that countless people carry in their bodies every day. God doesn't respond with anger and frustration to those who are triggered as they seek to clumsily take the journey of healing. He offers us mercy and comfort through His Spirit, therapy, community, and so much more.

These biological processes that happen deeply influence our emotional state, which affects our spiritual posture. Though we love to differentiate between the mind, body, and spirit, God created a beautifully intricate system where all three interact and affect each another.

AN INVITATION TO MORE

If there's anything I've learned through my work and personal life, it is that despite how painful triggers are, they are an invitation to more—to experience more of life, more of Jesus, more of ourselves, and more of the people God has entrusted us to.

Triggers remind us that we are carrying pain, even when we don't want to acknowledge it. They remind us that there is a part of us that is screaming to be seen, shouting through the pain via interruptions in our mood, inescapable patterns, unexplainable distance in our relationships, and dissatisfaction with our intimacy with God.

While we don't have control of our triggers, we do have control of what we do after we reflexively respond to the world around us. Without searching for the issues at the root of our patterns and responses, we get stuck in cycles of reactivity, like Tola. We feel on top of the world one minute and then like life isn't worth living the next.

Triggers remind us of the most wounded and fearful versions of ourselves. They bring up the emotions we are least acquainted with and expose us to thoughts and feelings that we spend most of our lives avoiding without even realizing it. They expose the reality of the feelings we'd experience if we didn't have our everyday dysfunctional patterns to protect us from our inner wounds. Triggers remind us that no matter how hard we work, no matter how many accolades we accumulate, we still carry the most vulnerable and terrified versions of ourselves wherever we go. And the parts of ourselves we so desperately want to silence and forget will make their way to the present at the most inconvenient times, if we don't hear what they have to say.

Whether we like it or not, the version of us that is revealed when we are triggered has a wisdom for the present that will allow us to live more fully. We can't control our triggers, but we can respond to them.

TRACE YOUR TRIGGERS

Think back to the negative core belief you have identified. As we build new patterns of reacting, we must know what type of moments are likely to elicit our negative emotional responses. You may notice that when your negative core belief and all the emotions tied to it are triggered, you act in a way that reflects the age at which your trauma first happened or was most impactful.

When we trace our triggers, we build the opportunity to gain understanding of why we react the way we do. This allows us to increase our empathy for ourselves and others as we journey toward healing and authenticity.

While thinking about your core negative belief, fill in these blanks below. This activity will allow you to simply see how your trauma (a moment from your ACE survey), negative core beliefs, negative patterns, and triggers all connect and feed into one another. When you answer honestly, these pointed moments can help you see how you engage with yourself and the world around you based on what you've experienced.

When we trace our triggers, we build the opportunity to gain understanding of why we react the way we do.

Wounding Moment (ACE Moment):

Life is:

I am (negative core belief):

I feel:

People are:

Relationships are:

I must (everyday patterns):

I need (everyday patterns):

I want (everyday patterns):

When I think of this moment, I feel the need to (triggering response):

While you complete these prompts, you may feel uncomfortable as sadness, anger, and other emotions attached to your patterns arise. The first time I completed this exercise, I cried, facing the truth of my unspoken but present perspectives. I finally saw how burdened I'd been. I also felt relief that those burdening perspectives finally had clear language.

Here's an example of how you can complete this activity:

Tola's Wounding Moment:

Being screamed at by her father for forgetting to complete a task

> **Life is:** unpredictable
> **I am:** in danger
> **I feel:** afraid
> **People are:** unsafe
> **Relationships are:** exhausting
> **I must:** be perfect, or I am in danger
> **I need:** freedom to be myself
> **I want:** to feel safe
> **When I think of this moment, I feel the need to:** make sure
>   everything is perfect, so no one will be upset with me

Because Tola decided to do the work of confronting her past and investigating her triggers, she began to see that she wasn't responsible for her father's joy or anger. Through our sessions, she began to investigate what her desires were apart from what she felt people would applaud her for. She began practicing how she would respond to people's disappointment, rather than seeking to avoid it altogether. She prioritized her emotional safety and began to take note of situations that triggered her. She began to give herself grace to step away from family trips that she knew she couldn't handle. Tola found that it wasn't possible for her to control the emotions of the people around her, but she could control how she treated herself and what environments she put herself in.

BEYOND THE SURFACE

Beneath the trigger is a version of yourself that you've only dreamed of. Not a perfect version of yourself, but a version that is free and loved. With every trigger, with every reactive response, God is leading you back to the moments at the core of your dysfunctional patterns, pointing to the times that defined your perception of your identity.

After being stuck in my own cycle of reactivity, which had me going from high motivation to crippling depression, I found myself in a time of prayer in my room. As I prayed, I got an image of myself coming to Jesus broken and battered. "I need a Band-Aid," I said to Him. He looked at me with tears in His eyes, then his eyes shifted downward to my stomach. When I looked down, my intestines were exposed, bloody, and oozing. In denial, I asked Him for another Band-Aid.

He looked at me with such tenderness and gently said, "No."

In the image, I screamed, thrashed, kicked, and hit as He embraced me. "No! No! No!" I screamed, intuiting that He wanted to care for my wound the way it needed to be cared for. He let me thrash for what felt like hours.

Finally, in exhaustion, I collapsed into His arms. I wept and wailed, and He hugged me tighter. "It's time," He said. "I have to clean it out. I know you are scared, but I'll give you courage. I'll be with you. It won't be easy; it won't be what you expect, but it will be beautiful. You won't believe what is on the other side."

Letting Jesus embrace us tangibly looks like acknowledging the true state of our hearts and minds and connecting to Him from the posture of the truth of where we are—and not where we want to be. It looks like discovering the tightly held beliefs we explored in our last activity, then prayerfully sharing those things with Jesus, the One who calls us friend. When we expose our wounded hearts to Him, we give Him the opportunity to heal, restore, and above all, comfort us in our brokenness.

He wants to revisit those moments and to heal them—to heal you. I know you might be scared. But He'll give you courage. It won't be what you expect, but in the end it will be beautiful.

Reflection Questions

1. What trauma response do you relate to most?
2. What triggering moment came up first when you completed the self-discovery activity?
3. What did it feel like to fill out these questions?
4. What did you learn about yourself through completing this activity?

chapter eight

GRIEVING THE LOSS:
WHAT DO I DO WITH THE PAIN?

I blacked out. When I woke up, my face was soaked with tears and six strangers were holding me tightly—some weeping with me and others holding back their tears with periodic sniffs. I was sweaty, shaking, and surrounded by a love I didn't know was real.

When I was six months pregnant, I attended the Onsite Leadership Academy retreat in the rolling hills near Nashville, Tennessee. Onsite is an incredible organization that provides mental health workshops to help people heal from deep wounds. The workshop I attended was specifically for mental health professionals, to help them identify and heal from the wounds that affect how they serve others in the field. Each of us was put in a group with six or seven other people. In the morning we had organizational trainings with the Onsite staff, and in the afternoons we gathered with our groups to engage in the mental health aspect of the workshop.

The time we spent together with our groups was intense,

eye-opening, and my first time participating in psychodrama—an experiential, action method of therapy and emotional healing, which allows you to act out scenarios you need to process so you can return to your pain and redeem the wounds of the past with the wisdom of the present.[1] We got the opportunity to spend time thinking and processing the personal moments of our lives that had become professional barriers. Then, one by one, we each brought our internal pains and struggles to the psychodramatic stage.

As others took their turns, I saw anger expressed in a way I had previously been told was unacceptable. There was a release of pain and an embrace of grief I had never witnessed before. I could see people being healed as they shouted the things they needed to say to people of their pasts, represented by people in the group. I got to play someone's mother, someone's sister, and someone's friend. I got to enter into people's experiences, increase my capacity for empathy, and also expand my view of how healing can be experienced.

When it was my turn to take center stage, I was terrified. I clammed up and shared a moment that frustrated me. But Jill, our facilitator, wouldn't let me get away with such a shallow attempt. "And what does that moment represent to you?" she asked.

My hands started shaking, and my eyes started watering; she knew based on bits and pieces I had shared earlier in group processing that there was more at the core of everything I had shared in that space. I knew, too, as I'd felt my body get hot in moments of expression, which I quenched with ice-cold shame.

Jill led me through speaking the truth of my anger, the truth of my frustration, the truth of my rage. I hated my trauma. I hated that I had to heal from it. I hated that healing was so hard. I hated that it affected every area of my life. In the throes of my psychodrama, I was consumed with rage. I felt so much shame. All my life I'd been taught anger was immaturity, anger was sin, anger was an indicator that you were out of God's will and far from Him.

"What are you feeling right now?" Jill asked. I didn't want to answer. The answer was obvious, and I felt like she was trying to embarrass me in a room full of people I didn't know.

"Anger," I whispered through tears.

"No," she quietly snapped back. "You feel rage." My cries became audible. I had felt so much rage for so many years. I felt trapped in it. No space ever allowed me to express it, and it compounded over time. I was ready to explode.

Every time I had tried to express my anger in the past, those around me were scared of it, embarrassed by it, or ashamed of it. I felt they were ashamed of me. I'd told myself if anyone saw my anger, they'd leave me, hate me, and drag my name through the dirt. It felt like my life depended on shutting this rage in, but I could feel it killing me.

That is not hyperbole. I regularly woke up in the middle of the night shaking. Sometimes I'd wake up with my fists balled up so tight that my nails would cut into the center of my palms, leaving bright-pink marks. My muscles were stiff. I had heart palpitations. I was quite literally being consumed by rage. I couldn't pray about it because everything I'd learned told me that being angry at, toward, or around God was irreverent. I didn't know what to do with my anger until that day.

"What does all emotion want to do?" Jill asked.

"I don't know," I responded through tears.

"All emotions want to move. E-motion. E-*motion*."

She walked over and handed me a bat with a padded end. I now know it's called a *bataka*. Then she dragged over a large, padded block that was three times the width of my body and about the height of my belly button. "Hit it," she said.

I lazily took a swat.

"No, no, no," she interrupted. "Keep your elbows in, bring it in over your head, and strike directly down." She physically moved me through the motion as she directed me. "Hit it."

I hit it with better form and more intensity.

"Again, harder." *Thwack!* I swung a little harder. "Again!" *Thwack!* I was gaining momentum.

I kept on hitting it, not needing her to tell me to do it anymore. With each strike, everything I shared with her and the group began to flash through my mind, as emotions coursed through my body. The betrayal, the dismissal, the abandonment, the abuse. I was feeling it all.

I hit the block harder and harder each time, my rage rising as I recalled all the moments that made me feel useless, all the people who made me feel shamed, all the pain that made me wonder whether living was worth it.

The room cheered as they celebrated my leaning into the exercise and letting my rage out. But at some point, the cheers stopped. Everyone grew silent, and the only sound in the room was the echo of the bataka slamming against the block, again and again and again. I let out a scream from the bottom of my belly. I roared until I ran out of breath, and I kept hitting that block. My rage was draining for the first time in my life. Once I felt it leaving, I couldn't stop. This was my chance to get it out—all the things I held in my body. This was my chance to get free, and I wasn't going to let it slip away. This was the only way.

I don't remember stopping. I just remember blinking like I had just woken up. I was sobbing. I sensed people around me. I had blacked out. As my vision focused, I realized I was being held by every person in my group. The heat of their bodies felt like a hug from God Himself.

I couldn't see Jill, but I could hear her.

"Kobe, this is how God responds to your rage when you dare to feel it in front of Him. He surrounds you. He holds you. You deserve to grieve. Bring your grief to Him."

There are many times when I've been surprised by God's response to my brokenness and pain, but to be honest, they felt relatively small and fleeting, especially in comparison to that moment. That day, I was overwhelmed with the tenderness Jesus offered me through the opportunity to be honest about my pain. It brought this scripture to mind:

> In my desperation I prayed, and the LORD listened;
> he saved me from all my troubles. (Psalm 34:6 NLT)

I felt seen. I realized that God made this space for me to feel, because He'd seen every burden I'd carried.

> You keep track of all my sorrows.
> You have collected all my tears in your bottle.
> You have recorded each one in your book. (Psalm 56:8 NLT)

I remembered that God sees the desires of my heart. He saw my longing to be free, and He gave me the opportunity to experience it.

> Praise the LORD, . . . who redeems your life from the pit
> and crowns you with love and compassion,
> who satisfies your desires with good things. (Psalm
> 103:2, 4–5)

HOW TO GRIEVE

I did not grow up in a world where I got to express my rage freely. I was often chastised about how I did it, when I did it, and who I did it around. I believed God cared more about how I expressed my emotions than He cared about the internal torture I lived through. As long as my pain didn't embarrass Him, I could express it; but if it did, there was no space for it. I'm so grateful God used the people at that retreat at Onsite to show me otherwise.

The pain of being awakened to how intensely and intimately our past wounds affect our present identity is brutal. The heartbreaking weight of seeing just how estranged we are from our authentic self and the love of God can invoke hopelessness in anyone. Emotions we were taught to never express or share rise to the surface of our lives as we become flooded with the reality of our complex, confusing, and painful past traumas.

After my clients recognize that their negative core beliefs and triggers reflect the deep, unaddressed wounds God wants to heal, they often ask, "What do I do now?"

My answer? You grieve.

The beginning of all healing is grieving. Grief is the anguish experienced after significant loss.[2] When we grieve, we acknowledge the great loss of safety, peace, assurance, acceptance, and so much more due to our trauma. Grieving requires that we look directly at what we have experienced and remember everything we didn't get, so we can allow ourselves to feel the full weight of the sadness we carry.

Most of us don't know how to grieve. We want a three-part, step-by-step formula. We want lifetime guarantees. We want to move on without getting close to the color, texture, tone, and temperature of our pain, not knowing that all healing comes from drawing near to brokenness, not running away from it. There's no restoration without grief. There is no healing without grief. There is no freedom without grief.

UNDERSTANDING EMOTIONS

Many of us have a poor understanding of what emotions are. We often want to exclude them from our experiences because we don't "get" them. We don't know where they fit into God's story and plan. We grew up hearing things like "Don't trust your feelings," or "It doesn't matter how you feel," from people who also taught us who God was and how to regard Him.

While well-meaning, many of these people missed the mark. In the midst of all the negative messages related to emotions, we've forgotten that emotions were created by God. There's a reason emotions are inextricable from any part of the human experience. There's a reason the absence of feelings and emotions is sickness. We don't reflect God's full image without emotions; we cannot live as we were designed to without emotions.

Emotions are neurological impulses that create physiological experiences as a response to personal appraisals of the world around us. With each emotion comes a specific secretion of hormones triggered by a stimulus. Emotions are meant to motivate us to action.

When we see a person steal something that is ours, our brain begins to appraise the situation, which is to simply develop an opinion or judgment about it. Once our brain receives information about the injustice, neurological impulses are created, which produce sensations that we experience and display in our bodies. If we get angry, we may feel hot, then ball up our fists. If we're sad, we may feel weight in our chest, then cross our arms. Even if we don't display our emotions through actions in our bodies, we still feel them in our bodies. If you take a look at the graphic below, you'll see just how each emotion registers in the body despite how it's physically expressed, which is usually based on our personalities, upbringing, and socialization.

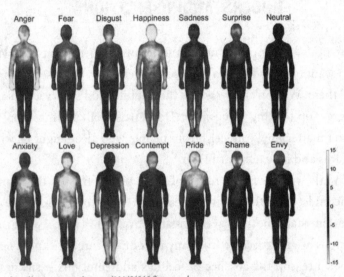

http://www.pnas.org/content/111/2/646.figures-only

Each appraisal is incredibly personal because it's based on our personal experiences. God truly made us all to be unique. What makes me angry may make my husband chuckle, and what annoys him to no end may be something I don't notice. Why? Because we've lived different lives, developed different values, and have different needs. Our emotions reflect the values and needs we have. And if we don't sit with them, we miss the opportunity to listen to what needs Jesus wants to fulfill in our lives.

Most of us don't know why certain emotions are communicated, so we try to shut them off. We want to stop feeling what we perceive as uncomfortable or even harmful. However, emotions cannot be selectively disregarded or turned off. Either they are all experienced fully, or they are not. We cannot have a deep and abiding relationship with the Lord (which Scripture often measures with emotions, such as joy) and then not feel despair in the presence of brokenness. Emotions are meant to assist us as we navigate the world and our relationship with God and humankind.

EMOTIONS AND THE CHURCH

We feel in our bodies, but trauma keeps many of us from becoming acquainted with our emotions. We don't want to feel or experience anything in our bodies due to traumas such as verbal abuse, bullying, or financial insecurity we experienced as children. But when we're estranged from our bodies, we remove ourselves from the sensations given to us by God to make sense of the world and experience His presence.

In church we often like to tell people to ignore their emotions, and I get why people say that. Sometimes you will have to persist and do things you don't want to do in the midst of uncomfortable feelings that won't go away. But to say you should ignore emotions altogether is just terrible for people's mental, emotional, and spiritual health. It confuses people when we make an appeal to their emotions, asking them to trust a God they can't see and to make a commitment that has eternal ramifications, just to turn right around and tell them not to trust their emotions.

We often miss the reality that many of us were originally drawn to God because of what we *felt*. We know this because we know that logic doesn't bring people to faith in Jesus but rather His Spirit does.

What we have received is not the spirit of the world, but the Spirit who is from God [the Holy Spirit], so that we may understand what God has freely given us. This is what we speak, not in words taught us by human wisdom but in words taught by the Spirit, explaining spiritual realities with Spirit-taught words. (1 Corinthians 2:12–13)

How do you sense God's Spirit in your life? I don't know many people who can answer that question without the word *feel*. I'm *not* saying that if we don't feel the Spirit, then He's not there. But I *am* saying that when we experience the Spirit, it is almost exclusively through emotions and the physical sensations that communicate them.

God designed the world and humankind masterfully. His intention for our creation is so magnificent that David wrote that we are fearfully and wonderfully made (Psalm 139:14). Yet in our culture and faith, we miss the intentionality of God's design when we bypass the reality that it was He who made emotions inextricable from the human experience. It was He who made it impossible to be healthily human and feel nothing at all. Yet we run from emotions, trying our best to scrub from our experiences the ones we don't understand, like scarlet letters that stain our humanity.

Emotions enhance our humanity and display our likeness to a beautifully infinite and deeply feeling God. But when we don't understand what emotions are for and what role they play in our lives, we can be overwhelmed by them or afraid to engage with them at all, touting them as sinful evidence that there's an enemy at work in our lives, rather than as evidence that there is a God who is relentless about our healing and wholeness even when we aren't.

The issue of trauma comes into play with our emotions when

we don't identify with them at all or overidentify with them. When we don't identify with our emotions, we are completely estranged from them and lose the ability to feel them deeply, name them, and be present with them. On the other hand, overidentifying with your emotions may look like being consumed by sadness to the point that you define yourself through the lens of it. It consumes you, as you have no tools for emotional regulation.

Because emotions are a response to external stimuli, our trauma makes our system of processing and receiving these stimuli disorganized, perceiving danger that elicits rage when we're safe, and safety that elicits joy when we're in danger. Just like in the garden of Eden, it inverts the original purpose of our emotions, taking the system that is meant to advocate for us and draw us closer to God and turning it into a system that leads us into more pain, heartbreak, and isolation.

Emotions enhance our humanity and display our likeness to a beautifully infinite and deeply feeling God.

Emotions, like every part of humanity, have been affected by the brokenness that has entered the world. But the original design of emotions is good. So when we let God restore our lives and restore our emotions, they can be one of the most powerful tools for connection, intimacy, and reconciliation. They help us experience liberation and life more abundantly.

Many people falsely equate a lack of emotions with spiritual maturity and higher levels of holiness. When we make that connection, we turn our backs on a Jesus who not only felt but also expressed a full range of emotions, yet remained holy. We turn our backs on a God who wept, overcome with such fear and anguish that blood seeped from His pores. We ignore a Jesus who cried over the death of His friend Lazarus just moments before He would raise him back to life. Stoicism is not holiness. Lack of empathy is not wisdom. Emotional repression is not health; it's unbiblical.

HOW TO FEEL

Akua (Ah-koo-ah) had a history of abuse and abandonment that deeply affected her everyday life. As we delved deeper into her trauma work, she would recall past moments that were tied to her present pain. But before she could share a glimpse of the burden she was carrying, she'd spend at least five minutes engaging in what I can only call a defense of her faith.

"I know that God is good, I know that I'm blessed, I know that other people would kill for the life I've had." She didn't realize it, but these weren't her words. She was rehearsing all the invalidating things she'd heard under the guise of spiritual encouragement. Her posture shriveled, and her face winced as she continued to put out all the phrases that had invalidated her real pain.

I gently interjected. "Can I jump in for a second?"

Her body jerked into the present as if she was just realizing where she was. She nodded slightly but didn't make eye contact. Shame was in the room. Shame from feeling too deeply, shame from trying to protect herself with the words that once battered her, shame that I noticed it all.

"I want you to close your eyes for a second," I said. She froze. I could tell she didn't know how to tell me she didn't feel safe closing her eyes. As she braced herself to power through, I leaned in and gently shared, "If you don't feel safe closing your eyes, feel free to soften your gaze and look into your lap or your hands. It's important that you feel safe as we do our work together. There will be a time in our work when pushing yourself to do things that make you feel uncomfortable will be good, but now isn't that time."

Her shoulders dropped with relief. She softened her gaze and looked down at her upturned palms. As I led her through deep breathing, I asked her to imagine that in her mind she could see her whole body. "As you hold that image in your mind, I want you to think of the physical sensation that you experience when you think about the abuse you've faced. Imagine that sensation is resting in a specific part of your body. Where would that be? And what color would it be?"

"My stomach, and it's bright red," she quickly responded.

"Okay, and what texture and temperature would that red sensation be?"

She took another breath. "It's hot like lava but sticky like putty."

Though she couldn't see me, I leaned in. "Mmm. I'm going to let you sit with that for about fifteen seconds."

Her eyes fluttered as they closed. I knew she was feeling deeply. Her fingers fidgeted as tears rolled down her face. I instructed her to take a deep breath, and I took one with her.

She opened her eyes. "Kobe, I'm angry. I'm angry that I had to experience that! I was just a kid, and I had no one to turn to. Everyone was so busy with their lives, no one even asked me if I was okay. They just spanked me and screamed at me for being 'disrespectful' and not listening. Every time I tried to tell someone when I got older, I couldn't even get through sharing how I felt without them shutting me down with Scripture."

She cried as she talked with her hands and from her heart. "Now I don't even know how to trust God. I feel like He's angry at me for being angry like everyone else." As she sobbed unconsolably, I silently scooted my chair closer to her. Her hand quickly darted out and grabbed my right hand. I gave it a squeeze and gently placed my left hand on top of hers, soaking in the courage it took for her to reach out and wade in the sea of grief she'd been drowning in.

Today though, the waters were still raging, and she caught a breath she'd been gasping for, for years.

EXPERIENCING OUR EMOTIONS

When we allow ourselves to experience the emotions that arise as we grieve, we gain access to the stories of sadness, anger, and disappointment that we've held on to. These are stories that need to be heard. Without our knowing these stories and becoming acquainted with the needs that we have, these needs can't get met. What we feel *can* be healed. To resolve the circuitry of being trapped and held hostage by emotions, these emotions have to be named and experienced in our bodies.

We grieve to experience the truth of where we are, even when it's painful. We grieve because our expressions of pain are vulnerable worship to God. We grieve because it frees us from the illusion of control and allows us to fix our eyes on the One who is our refuge. Here are some tangible ways we can begin our journey of grieving.

Movement

Movement is a powerful way to grieve. It requires us to notice how the issues of our hearts show up in our bodies so that we can respond in the ways we need. My experience at Onsite is a glimpse into how movement is important to the healing process. The accumulation of cortisol and adrenaline, on top of having a dysregulated nervous system, kept me physically and emotionally hostage.[3] Even as I avoided looking at what broke my heart, it didn't change that those same emotions I ignored controlled my life. Freedom and healing came from the movement of swinging the bat during our exercise. It came from acknowledging the wholistic loss that comes from abuse, which affects the mind, body, and soul. It's important to tell our story with our words, but we can't forget that our bodies have stories to tell too.

Movements like slow and mindful stretching, dancing, walking, and skipping can help us grieve as we allow the pent-up emotions we've carried to be released from our bodies. Intentional movement communicates to our fear-based circuits to decrease activity—allowing space for safety, spontaneity, and creativity. Movement allows us to express the accumulated energy the body has gathered through the physical effects of trauma.

Name It to Tame It

World-renowned psychiatrist Dr. Dan Siegel coined the term "name it to tame it"—a psychological and neurological principle which communicates that when we label our feelings, we decrease the stress we experience.[4] When we put words to what we are carrying, we experience our emotions as less painful and overwhelming.

We can activate the "name it to tame it" principle through prayer, journaling, songwriting, speaking, singing, and any form of expression that allows us to move through the emotions about which we often feel stuck utilizing words.

Breath Prayer

The breath prayer is a powerful, ancient Christian spiritual discipline that allows us to connect to God by presenting intimate desires through prayers, utilizing our breath. This grief practice is especially powerful for those of us who may feel overwhelmed, frustrated, sad, or distant from God.[5]

- As you inhale and as your stomach expands, repeat a simple, one-sentence prayer that begins with calling on a name or quality of God.
- Then as you exhale, as your stomach deflates, share a phrase that reflects a deep desire you want to acknowledge before God, or a truth you want Him to settle in your soul.

This is a powerful way to invite God into the physical experience of your pain, through slowing your breath and regulating your nervous system. It also activates the "name it to tame it" principle as you use your words to invite the Holy Spirit to respond to the wholistic experience of your pain. Here are some examples of breath prayers:

> *Inhale: Good God,*
> *Exhale: my pain matters to You.*
> *Inhale: Father,*
> *Exhale: I am safe with You.*
> *Inhale: Jesus,*
> *Exhale: You see my broken heart.*
> *Inhale: Abba,*
> *Exhale: show me You care.*

Lament

Lamenting is a spiritual discipline that allows us to invite God into our experiences of grief through five key elements:

Address to God: calling on Him in a way that is authentic to you

Complaint: telling God what is making you frustrated

Request: asking for God's help to do something about it

Motivation: explaining to God why He should be motivated to do this

Confidence: communicating what you know of God that empowers you to have faith

Lamenting is a practice that is powerfully displayed in songwriting, poetry, and journaling. It allows us to acknowledge our pain and experience the emotions tied to the pain by becoming acquainted with how our experiences affect us and then inviting God into our experience of pain. Lament reminds us that we're not alone, that it's good to feel, and that healing comes from engaging with our pain instead of avoiding it.

THE BEGINNING OF RESTORATION

Grieving is the first step of healing and restoration. It's where we see the full landscape of our pain and bring it to Jesus. Healing is not about forgetting the past; it's about experiencing the redemption of past moments that traumatize us in the present. It's about the restoration of our most authentic selves in Christ as we reclaim everything He designed us to experience before we were wounded.

It's about coming home to Jesus, to ourselves, and to the liberation He died for us to experience.

Before we can be restored, we have to recognize what was lost. Feeling and connecting to our emotions gives us the valuable information we need for healing. It gives us the opportunity to experience the divine comfort of the Holy Spirit. If we're always consoling ourselves, when does God get a chance to be our comforter? As we let God and others show up for us, we gain the courage to show up for ourselves in the ways we deserved but didn't experience.

Mourning is the beautiful acknowledgement of how trauma turned our world upside down. It is acknowledging the safety we didn't get, the love we longed for, the intimacy that we struggled to grasp. It's a reminder of why the greatest gift Jesus left the entire world was His Spirit, whom He called "the Comforter" (John 14:26 KJV). Our deep wounds need divine presence. Grieving gives us access to that presence. When we pretend our pain isn't that bad, we forfeit the supernatural comfort God wants to give us. When we lean in to honest presence with Jesus, it reflects the actions we take in faith as we believe that He sees our pain—and that He'll be moved to do something about it.

When we access our emotions, we access the messages they are trying to tell us. Connecting to our emotions allows us to utilize the system of awareness, connection, and appraisal that God has given us to help deal with the hardships of life. When Akua began to grieve what she had experienced, she created room for new messages and perspectives to settle her heart. She was no longer consumed by sadness. She made space to feel the weight of what she didn't get and what she should have gotten, so that when she does receive what she needs now, she can do so with joy.

For those of us who've spent our lives stuck in patterns of acting, defending, and pretending to be okay while enduring deep pain, the fullness of our grief is where we'll find the fullness of God's love for us. When we are at our weakest, when we finally face how broken we really are and how little power we have to be or do anything for ourselves or others, we're faced with a desperate need that causes us to cry out for more. We want Jesus. The One who is strong in our weakness, the One who has compassion on the brokenhearted, the One who walks up to people and heals them before they do a thing for Him.

Feeling and connecting to our emotions gives us the valuable information we need for healing.

I was there in that moment I described at the beginning of this chapter—releasing my rage through psychodrama at Onsite. I needed Jesus then and still do. I couldn't go on living without Him. The pain of life was too heavy, too complex, too demanding, and I needed rest, but there was none to be found in the flesh. I didn't need a master to serve. I was the lost sheep. Alone, confused, disoriented, with no sense of direction, with no idea where home was, I needed a shepherd to find me and guide me home. I needed a father running to me with arms wide-open. That's what I got.

Surrounded by strangers, on the floor of a cold room in Tennessee, I mourned for the first time in years. I opened the door to a part of my heart I had kept locked. The pain was more than I anticipated, the grief was heavier than I could bear. But the tenderness Jesus showed me through those strangers, many of whom were not believers, was and is something that brings me to tears, even as I write this. I had no clue that type of acceptance existed. I screamed as loud as I could and beat an inanimate object with a rage that overwhelmed my body. I was supposed to be shamed, I was supposed to be laughed at, my faith was supposed to be brought into question, my professionality was supposed to be challenged—but instead I was held. Like a child drawn in by a loving parent, I was cradled in the arms of people I didn't know. And I was reminded of a love I'd forgotten about in Jesus.

Grieve with Jesus. Invite Him into your pain through movement, breath prayer, and lamenting. Speak the emotions you feel in your body. Bring your pain to Him and lay it at His feet. Tell Him how you feel; share what breaks your heart. It already breaks His.

As you seek to transform yourself every day and to heal from the trauma of your past, know every emotion you bring to Him can and will be touched by Him. The tenderness that He will give you is what will keep you from running back to the same patterns that draw you away from freedom and into darkness. When we dare to feel and grieve, we gain access to the divine comfort and presence of God.

Reflection Questions

1. What did your trauma keep you from receiving?
2. What activity listed in this chapter are you most drawn to, to help you grieve?
3. What emotions are you feeling that you can express to God in that activity?

chapter nine

MOVING FORWARD:
HOW DO I BEGIN HEALING?

The book of Exodus recounts when God liberated the Israelites from the enslavement and oppression of the Egyptian empire. We learn about the final moments when the Israelites escaped the bonds of slavery. After more than four hundred years of working seven days a week with no rest and no breaks, they were finally able to leave Egypt and journey toward the promised land—the home God promised to Israel through Abraham.

As they journeyed through the desert to their destination, the Israelites began to complain. It was taking longer and was harder than they expected. Though they longed for freedom, they were nervous about the unknown life outside of slavery. They struggled to depend on God and found themselves grumbling about how they would have been better off remaining enslaved.

I know we often give the Israelites a hard time because of their impatient behavior. But here's something to think about: *we* are the Israelites, struggling to find healing in our lives.

We so desperately want freedom, but when we get it, it's hard to exist in. The distance between us and the painful moments of our lives didn't change as much as we hoped it would. Some of us are accustomed to the slavery of terror and pain we hate so much. The repetition of fear we've lived in has wired our brains to default to emotional postures that keep us from seeing that there is promise for us in the journey.

When we are out of the immediate pain of the traumas we've endured, the shock of living presently can be jarring. We find that all we asked for is not all we dreamed of. The unpredictability of relying on God in a new way feels unnatural and scary for those of us who have been mindlessly floating through life just trying to survive.

The Israelites grumbled of hunger, as they feared that God wouldn't meet their needs. But in true God fashion, He said these words, "I have heard the complaints of the Israelites. So tell them, 'Tonight you will eat meat. And in the morning you will have all the bread you want. Then you will know you can trust the LORD, your God'" (Exodus 16:12 ERV).

God didn't shame His people for not trusting Him; He simply showed Himself to be trustworthy. He did this for them because He's loving. He does this for us today because He's still loving.

God continued to provide the Israelites with food throughout their trek. But He also gave them clear instructions on how to collect and store it, so they could honor the Sabbath—the day of rest that was meant to be a gift to a people who, for four hundred years, had no rest. Instead, some of the Israelites gathered more food than needed. The issue wasn't their inability to trust God; it was the idea of scarcity that four hundred years of slavery had created in them. The posture of scarcity kept them from trusting in the gift of God's provision; it kept them from honoring the rest He wanted to restore.

The reality of the brokenness of the Israelites was laid bare in the desert. God spent about forty days getting them out of Egypt, but it took forty years in the desert to get Egypt out of them. I imagine God knew that the promised land He was calling them to would be so much sweeter a gift if they weren't in bondage.

Sometimes it's not until we get everything we want that we realize it's not the changes in our external environment that needed attention; it's our internal landscape that needs restoration.

When we get friends but still feel lonely, friendship isn't the problem. When we get the job but still feel empty, the job isn't the problem. When we get fame, fortune, and notoriety but still feel skeptical, afraid, and mistrusting of whether we're loved and cared for, there is work that still needs to be done.

It's not the things; it's the heart.

The Israelites got everything they'd been longing for—complete freedom from oppression. Yet they couldn't enjoy it; they couldn't receive it. Their hearts had to be changed and healed before they could receive the gift of the promised land they were headed to. The desert was their journey of healing, where they dwelled with and depended on God. He is inviting you into childlike reliance and trust in Him, just as He did for the Israelites. He's initiating your freedom with moments that will help you venture into the untouched landscape of your heart.

In the desert, God began healing the Israelites of each of the values and principles they adopted in slavery. He did this by calling them to a series of actions and inactions that reflected and embodied the very opposite of what they'd neurologically been conditioned to do.

They were conditioned to hoard, for fear of scarcity.

They were conditioned to forecast for tomorrow, rather than enjoy today.

They were conditioned to find safety in predictability, rather than in the character of God.

With each action, God sought to change their hearts, rewire their brains, and set their souls on their true hope and security: Him. And in Him, they would be reminded of the calling they had to one another and to the world. To the unsuspecting eye, the only issue with the Israelites was that they were enslaved, but when God removed them from slavery, it exposed all the issues beneath the surface.

When it feels too hard to change, know that God created our brains with the power of neuroplasticity, the ability to create new connections and create new patterns. We've learned new things once and we can learn new things again. There will be discomfort, but discomfort is a sign of change, not a signal to stop. When acting in opposition to what you've always believed feels awkward and uncomfortable, remind yourself that discomfort is a sign of change. You are changing.

When we begin to heal our traumatic wounds, we start to act in alignment with something other than the lies we've believed, even when we still believe them. That looks like reaching out to a trusted friend when you'd rather not share about your depressive episode. It may look like seeking therapy when you're used to powering through your anxiety or finding ways to distract from it altogether. It may also mean speaking up and allowing yourself to be center stage when you feel like God has given you something to say, rather than cowering in fearful shame. And for some of us, it means resting in silence as we choose not to fight battles that aren't ours.

God is calling us to something different. He's calling us to oppose our status quo with actions that align with the truth of who we are and to practice healing until we can feel it. God is calling us to rely on Him and to trust who He says we are and live as He's called us to live.

THE PATH OF HEALING

"I don't even know who I am anymore."

I've said these words so many times in the last few years. I've heard these words even more as a therapist. These words have been spoken through rage, tears, laughter, relief, and frustration. Every person recovering from trauma gets to this place at some point—the place where they become painfully aware of how much of their life has nothing to do with living in their authentic identity and so much to do with coping with and distracting from pain.

After the patterns have been explained, trauma has been unveiled, the negative core beliefs have been revealed, the terror has been exposed, and the triggers have been explained, it's easy to wonder what's left beneath the rubble of the life we once knew. For those of us who wanted simple behavioral changes, the path of trauma recovery we ended up on feels like going to the doctor for a checkup only to end up in surgery.

The whirlwind of past pain we have faced leaves us asking,

What happens next?
What is God going to do about what He brought up?
How will He restore this?
What will restoration look like when I've lost so much of what I
  thought was my identity?

Sometimes we can be so consumed with healing that we don't care about the actual healing; we just want to appear healed so we can escape the vulnerability of being seen in our brokenness in front of other people. If there's one thing you leave this book with, I want it to be this: healing is not the goal; it's the byproduct. I've found that healing is a cyclical journey of focusing on four things: boundaries, acceptance, courage, and connection. When we make these things foundational parts of our lives, we can walk the lifelong journey of healing without feeling overwhelmed.

Boundaries require that we utilize our understanding of our emotions to gauge how close we can be to others, while honoring our needs and remaining authentic. Acceptance allows us to unashamedly address the truth of what we're experiencing, without feeling the burden to pretend like we are somewhere else. Acceptance helps us pursue change because of love, rather than out of hate. Courage helps us use God's tenderness and care toward us as fuel to approach new things with childlike faith. Connection to safe and trustworthy people reminds us that we are worthy of love and attention, no matter what emotional state we are in. Healing is a journey, not a destination. We can work through all the pain in the world, but we have no clue how our past pain will interact with it.

I've been taught in so many ways that healing is fervent, hour-long prayer that casts out demons while speaking in tongues. It was always communicated with words or actions that healing was about trying harder, being more disciplined, making myself consistently do the things I struggled to do minute by minute. This created a cycle of trying as hard as I could to please God with 5:00 a.m. prayers, strict fasting, and never missing a church service. But when I got too weary, I was back in the pit of despair, stuck in a hole with my brokenness.

Connection to safe and trustworthy people reminds us that we are worthy of love and attention, no matter what emotional state we are in.

When we focus on what we can allow ourselves to experience in our brokenness, rather than what we will demand of ourselves, we begin to live sustainably in the path of restoration. Further burdening ourselves to make our pain go away doesn't work. Working to prove our worthiness harms us more. If my hard work was the only thing that could give me access to God's healing power, I'd never experience healing.

Thankfully, there is a better way.

TAKE THE LEAP

Take a second to think back to your negative core belief. Notice what emotions you feel and where you feel them in your body. Write it down if you can.

Now I want you to answer this question: What is the exact opposite belief—your positive core belief? If your belief is *I am shameful*, the opposite of that belief could be *I am good as I am* or *I am worthy of honor*. If your belief is *I am bad*, your positive core belief would be *I am good*.

Whatever your new positive core belief is, I want you to sit with it and imagine what it would be like to wake up on most days and believe this is 100 percent true. What emotion does that bring up for you? Where does it come up in your body? What everyday choices would you make? What would your life look like?

Envision a future resting in your positive core belief system. I've created a list to guide you through discovering what your positive core belief may be. This list isn't exhaustive; you may have a belief that isn't listed, and that's okay. You may notice that some positive core beliefs are listed more than once (e.g., I am lovable). That's completely normal. It's common for differing negative core beliefs to have identical positive core beliefs.

Positive Core Belief Checklist

Survival

- ☐ I can survive
- ☐ I can have my needs met
- ☐ I deserve to exist

Shame (I am wrong)

- ☐ I am okay as I am
- ☐ I can accept myself
- ☐ I am good enough the way I am
- ☐ I can recognize appropriate responsibility
- ☐ I am not defined by my mistakes
- ☐ I am not defined by what I've been through
- ☐ I am lovable
- ☐ I am good
- ☐ I am lovable
- ☐ My body is good
- ☐ I deserve good things
- ☐ I am valuable
- ☐ I am enough
- ☐ I belong
- ☐ I am beautiful

- ☐ I am intelligent

Worth/Lovability

- ☐ I am lovable
- ☐ I am worthy
- ☐ I am acceptable as I am
- ☐ I am lovable
- ☐ I am wanted by the right people
- ☐ There are people who love me
- ☐ I bring value to people and places
- ☐ I will be accepted by people who value me
- ☐ I am loved

Guilt (I've done something wrong)

- ☐ I can learn from my mistakes
- ☐ I did what I could with what I had

Safety/Vulnerability

- ☐ I can be trustworthy
- ☐ I can learn to trust myself
- ☐ I can learn to trust my judgment

- ☐ I can learn to trust the right people
- ☐ I have the resources to protect myself
- ☐ I am safe
- ☐ It's okay to show and express my emotions
- ☐ I can stand up for myself

- ☐ I am enough
- ☐ I am effective at what I'm resourced to do
- ☐ I can trust the right people
- ☐ I am able to change
- ☐ I can protect myself when I have the ability to exercise control

Control/Choice

- ☐ I can recognize what I can and can't control
- ☐ I can control what I can
- ☐ I have great strengths
- ☐ I can safely let go of some control
- ☐ I can control what I can even when . . .
- ☐ I am capable
- ☐ I can succeed
- ☐ I am able to make choices to change my life
- ☐ I do not have to be perfect to be loved

Capability

- ☐ I am not helpless
- ☐ I have power and control over certain areas of life
- ☐ I can demonstrate strength
- ☐ I can rely on myself and my strengths
- ☐ I can handle important things
- ☐ I am competent

Toxic/Shame

- ☐ I deserve to exist

While you stayed with the thought of what your life could look like if you believed differently about yourself, you may have (even if it was just for a moment) felt an emotion associated with that positive core belief. Was it a flash of hope? A trickle of joy? Budding laughter? Our holy imagination from God allows us to look forward with joyful anticipation rather than with fear. The only difference between anxiousness and excitement is whether we're anticipating the good or the bad. We can't magically change how our bodies respond, but we can use its natural processes in our favor.

What if God is calling you to make one new decision a day that reflects the version of yourself that embodies your positive core belief? Positive core beliefs reflect the version of you that feels free. What if He's calling you to something as simple as taking lunch breaks instead of powering through the workday? Or resting because you're tired, not because you've earned it? Maybe He's inviting you into a hobby that doesn't earn you money or demand productivity. God is calling you to the risk of doing something new. Many of us are unaccustomed to living life outside of our pain, just like the Israelites, who were unaccustomed to living life outside of slavery. Though we long to be free from it, we don't know how to exist outside of it. Taking these small steps teaches us how.

Before we can jump into taking these risks, we first have to address the key barriers that keep us from being courageous and trying new and different things: our automatic negative thoughts.

AUTOMATIC NEGATIVE THOUGHTS

Automatic negative thoughts (ANTs) are defined as negative thoughts "that are instantaneous, habitual, and nonconscious." They affect a person's mood and actions by releasing hormones that induce sadness, anger, shame, and more.[1] The feelings that accompany automatic negative thoughts then create a cycle where our responses validate the original negative thoughts. Maybe this is why Scripture tells us to think on what is good, pure, noble, admirable, excellent, and praiseworthy (Philippians 4:8). Our thoughts truly do have so much power. For people who've endured trauma, this feels like an almost impossible task. Without addressing our thoughts, the negative cycle feeds itself.

We interrupt the cycle of automatic negative thinking by killing the ANTs. Coined by psychiatrist Dr. Daniel Amen, "Killing the ANTs" explains how we can interact with the automatic negative thoughts that arise from the past traumatic experiences we've endured. The activity below is adapted from his practice and work.[2]

How to Kill the ANTs

1. Write down the automatic negative thoughts that come from your negative core belief. Mine would be "No one really likes me," since I often believe that I am bad.

2. Identify the ANT species. There are nine types of ANTs.

   - All-or-Nothing ANTs: Thinking that things are either all good or all bad
   - Less-Than ANTs: Comparing and seeing yourself as less than others
   - Just-the-Bad ANTs: Seeing only the bad in a situation
   - Guilt-Beating ANTs: Thinking in words like *should*, *must*, *ought*, or *have to*
   - Labeling ANTs: Attaching a negative label to yourself or someone else
   - Fortune-Telling ANTs: Predicting the worst possible outcome for a situation with little or no evidence for it
   - Mind-Reading ANTs: Believing you know what other people are thinking even though they haven't told you
   - If-Only and I'll-Be-Happy-When ANTs: Arguing with the past and longing for the future
   - Blaming ANTs: Blaming someone else for your problems

3. Ask yourself, *Is this thought 100 percent true?*
   - How do you feel when you have this thought?
   - How do you act when you have this thought?
   - What is the outcome of those actions?
   - How would you feel without this thought?[3]

DEVELOPING HOPE FOR NEW PATTERNS

Now I want you to think about what it would be like to wake up most days and believe that your positive core belief is 100 percent true. As you do this, answer the questions below.

1. How would you feel if you believed this were true?
2. Where would you experience that feeling in your body?
3. How would you act if you had this positive thought?
4. What would the outcome of these actions be in your everyday life?

What is one small action you can take to reflect the truth of your positive core belief? Can you do that today? Can you commit to doing it once a week? Start small. It's okay to start with sparse, inconsistent change. Consistency comes from confidence. Allow yourself to build confidence in breaking the cycles you've been stuck in, before you step into whole-life changes. God is inviting you into new patterns, to reflect the new life that's ahead of you.

I remember needing to buy a pair of jeans after my last pair ripped. I sat on my couch with an order of jeans in my online cart for two hours. I couldn't click "check out." My negative core belief was at work even in the small and seemingly insignificant things, like buying a pair of jeans. When I built up the courage to continue checking out, I cried.

"I deserve to have my needs met," I said to myself. To many people, this moment was small and laughable, but for me it was the seed of a monumental shift taking place in my heart. *I fought the lie.* I kept in sight the truth of who I am now—even though I didn't feel it—and I did something I usually wouldn't have done. I created a new neurological pathway. I opened my brain and my heart to new possibilities.

This is what doing the work of trauma looks like. It's often our daily unseen patterns that break the generational cycles passed down to us, and rarely the grand gestures we perform in front of an audience.

Someone once said our actions become our habits and our habits become our character. I've seen that to be true time and time again. We break cycles by allowing ourselves to experience tenderness and love. We allow that love to become our key motivation because, when it is, we feel safe enough to try something different. Something that reflects who we are and not what we're afraid of, because the patterns of our heart and mind have been changed long before we tried to break the pattern of our actions. When we experience the taste of freedom and acceptance that's present when we fail *and* when we succeed, we find a home with ourselves and God. We experience healing that doesn't come from being perfect but from loving every version of ourselves that survived heartache.

We break cycles by allowing ourselves to experience tenderness and love.

LOVING YOURSELF

God longs for us to love ourselves. He wants us to live out of our positive core beliefs. When it comes to this part of healing, many of my Christian clients struggle to lean in to the idea of self-love. "The heart of man is evil and there is no good in it!" they will say, or "I'm not called to love myself; I'm called to love others!" They mistake self-loathing for righteousness and think their self-deprecating behavior will garner favor for them in heaven. Though they rarely say it, they desperately want to feel at home in their own bodies, find joy in who they are, and live free and abundant lives. But often, Christians have been taught that to love themselves is to deny the gospel and betray the sacrifice of Jesus Christ. The dissonance between what their soul craves and what they've been taught is "good" is excruciating.

Nneka (Neh-kah) was a client who came to see me specifically for religious trauma. She struggled with recurring depressive episodes, suicidal thoughts, and low self-esteem. She felt like developing love for herself was sinful and was therefore resistant to therapeutic interventions that would make her better, even though she hated being depressed.

"Are we called to love what God loves?" I asked her in one session.

"Of course!" she exclaimed.

"Do you think Jesus loves you?"

"Yes! I do," she continued.

"So how can you hate what He loves?"

She sat silently as she began to open herself to the idea that hating herself wasn't an act of holiness. She had spent years denying her needs of safety and belonging, ignoring her desires to leave an abusive church and marriage, and taking up a cross that God hadn't given her.

"But Scripture tells us to be humble," she replied, in a last-ditch effort to protect her own oppression.

"Do you know what the biblical definition of humble is?"

She shook her head.

I went on to explain to her that many people believe the word "humility" in Scripture can be defined as "believing you are who God says you are." God calls Israel royal diadems and crowns of splendor, a royal priesthood, and a reflection of His very image.

God doesn't delight in our self-hatred. To love ourselves is to love God; to hate ourselves is to hate His very image. God wants us to see the wonder and delight in ourselves that He sees in us. He wants us to live joyful lives of abundance and longs to satisfy our desires with good things. He crowns us with love and compassion, with attentive care that moves Him to action. This is the action that He is moved to: to restore the joy of our souls by restoring the joy of our identity. When we want more of life, He doesn't close His fist and pull away; He pours out more of Himself—more tenderness, more compassion, more peace.

Will there be hardship? Absolutely. Will there be heartache? Without a doubt. Will you need to make hard sacrifices? Yes. But are our lives called to be defined by the hardship we endure or by the goodness of God we experience? I'll let you answer that for yourself.

If you're still struggling to find your footing in who you are as you stand between the trauma of the past and the promise of the future, here is your answer: you are Abba's child. You are a reflection of God's wisdom, joy, creativity, peace, love, kindness, compassion, and justice. Every excited inkling you have to call a friend is part of His attentiveness. Every dream you have to give generously to others is a call to the spirit of generosity He placed in you.

You are a royal diadem—a crown of splendor. You are the apple of His eye, the child He's proud of, the child He loves to dwell with, the child He loves to bless.

You are not defined by what happened to you—even when you feel like it. Read your positive core belief. This is what God believes about you. Say it out loud. This is what God says about you.

The tenderness of Jesus exposes us to our most salient identity. In Him we get to experience the very antithesis of our negative core beliefs. Those who carry shame receive acceptance, and the hopeless begin to dream again.

I'm not telling you to say this out loud because of some arbitrary idea. I say this because we are actually using the very systems that our brains used against us in trauma, for our benefit.

So many of us heard, saw, and experienced wounding events over and over again. The repetition of these events created well-versed neurological pathways that made it easier for our brains to believe those things about ourselves than the things that are true. When we repeat the positive truth of who we are, even when our emotions are in complete contrast to that negative identity, we are building new neurological pathways related to the truth of who we are. This new cycle reflects the truth of Proverbs 18:21, "The tongue has the power of life and death, and those who love it will eat its fruit."

Why? Because we will believe most intensely what we hear most often.

When we speak these truths about ourselves and place ourselves in an environment and around people who also believe this, we embody the word of the Lord through Ezekiel: "Prophesy to these bones and say to them, 'Dry bones, hear the word of the LORD! This is what the Sovereign LORD says to these bones: I will make breath enter you, and you will come to life.'" (Ezekiel 37:4–5).

God is restoring who you see yourself to be. He is directly refuting, again and again, the negative core beliefs that keep showing up, the beliefs that keep you shackled to fear even when you're striving toward the purpose you know God has called you to. He's inviting you to take the leap and act on something you don't believe—to build new patterns, shaped by a heavenly reality that you will one day live in if you just jump, if you dare to lean in to something you can't yet feel even if you can sense it.

It will be hard. It might feel terrifying. You'll be fighting the emotions of the past as you make new choices for your future. Just like the Israelites, you'll want to turn back. The uncertainty may feel overwhelming, the intimacy may feel terrifying, and you may find yourself wishing for the very things you prayed to be healed and saved from. On some days the tenderness of Jesus will calm the storm, and on others you'll feel out of control, when it seems like Jesus is sleeping as the storm rages. Either way, His presence will be there.

The journey is long, but the presence of God in it is beautiful, tangible, and what really keeps us going. Some days, you'll trek forward as the presence of the Lord leads you with clouds; other nights, you'll journey through the darkness as God leads you with a pillar of fire. At times, you'll rest with Him, not moving at all as He dwells with you, making your heart His tent of meeting. His tenderness will be your source; without it you won't be able to keep going.

Nneka struggled to stay close to a God she felt was perpetually disappointed in her. A God who delighted in her self-loathing, instead of one who freed her from it. During our time working together, she began to develop a perspective of God that was rooted in His delight in her, regardless of what she did or didn't do. Nneka found herself wanting to be honest with God and wanting to love herself through boundaries. She began to develop a love for herself that reflected the love God has for her.

Many of us have been told in one way or another that if something is hard, it's a sign that we shouldn't be doing it. We've been told that all good things that are for us are meant to come easily. I don't believe in that sentiment at all. Sometimes when even the simplest things are hard, it is evidence that we are doing divine work—warring against unseen opposition and fighting for something that will change our lives and every life God will connect us to.

To experience the change, to see the transformation, we have to rest in His tenderness and take risks that refute the lies in our hearts.

Reflection Questions

1. Write down your negative core beliefs and your positive core beliefs.
2. Complete the "Kill the ANTs" activity with some of the thoughts that arise when you believe that your negative core belief is true.

chapter ten

TRUSTING OTHERS WITH MY PAIN: WHAT IF I CAN'T DO IT ALONE?

I felt the Holy Spirit while jamming out to a Justin Bieber song on my way to class. I was making my weekly commute between Wilmington and Charlotte, North Carolina. Though I lived in Wilmington, I was attending seminary at Gordon-Conwell and needed to be there weekly.

The commute was brutal. After working two internships and a job, I would get in the car on Fridays, drive four hours to Charlotte, clean myself up in a Chick-fil-A bathroom, and head to class that evening. Then I'd wake up early on Saturday for class the entire day before making the four-hour drive back to Wilmington. I did this almost every weekend for three years, and for a portion of that time, I was pregnant. It wore me down in ways I can't explain.

One day as I drove on a long stretch of Interstate 85, my mind began to wander. I started to think about the life I had in contrast to the life I felt like I was created for. I love to sing, to dance, and to experience thrill-filled adventure, but I couldn't remember the last time I had sung in the shower, danced to my favorite song, or tried something new.

I felt like I had to wait to be happy. I felt like life had to get easier and things had to be more orderly before I could start doing the things I loved again. I felt like I needed to push through the healing, so I could get to the "good part" of life when my trauma would be a thing of the past and I could live freely.

Even though I felt that way, everything I knew about healing urged me not to give in to that notion. So, at 12:45 p.m. on my way to Charlotte, I busted out in the most elaborate (and driver-safe) arm choreography you've ever seen a person do. I danced until I laughed. I laughed until I cried. I hadn't moved my body in so long. I could feel the stress, tension, and anxiety leaving my body. This was healing—for my mind, body, and soul.

Most of us believe the myth that we have to put our lives on hold to heal. The truth is, healing happens *as* we live. As we take the steps, as we try the new things. Healing is a heart posture. It's a journey, not a destination. Healing happens in the everyday moments and patterns of life, not in the margins of it.

As I danced in the midst of so much stress, I was reminded that two things can be true: life can be hard, *and* I can still have fun. I can feel anxious *and* try new things. I can experience sadness *and* still treat myself with love. I felt the presence of God in the most unexpected place. In the risk of trying something new and denying the lies in my head, God comforted me. I was covered in goose bumps that seemed to communicate, "Dance, girl, dance! That's what I'm talking about!"

Healing isn't just bitter tears and heart-wrenching prayers. Healing is about restoring the freedom that was lost. It's about laughing until your stomach hurts, reminding yourself that you *can* focus on joy. It's about dancing around the house as you demand nothing of your body, teaching yourself that the abuse you experienced in your body doesn't define its purpose or worth. Healing is also lighthearted and soft moments. It's making safety a priority, even when others don't understand it. It's speaking well of yourself and not turning down compliments. Healing is connecting deeply to others and trying new things. It's engaging in creativity and spontaneity as you relearn freedom.

Healing happens in the everyday moments and patterns of life, not in the margins of it.

YOU HAVE TO GET IT OUT

Healing from our deepest wounds requires that we acknowledge them. Not just in our hearts but with our words. Have you ever wondered if you really need to talk about it over and over again? The answer to that is yes. And if you've said in the silence of your heart, *I'm so tired of talking about this; I just want to be over it,* though you may not feel it, you're in one of the best places you can be.

Some of us know that the burning in our hearts and the churning in our stomachs signal that we need to speak up. It's a visceral experience that seems to be universal. God wants us to talk about what we've experienced because He wants healing for us. Speaking about it sets us on the path of restoration and redemption both spiritually and biologically.

Earlier we spoke about Dr. Dan Siegel and the principle he coined: name it to tame it.[1] This phrase reflects his neurological research, which found that when we feel distressing emotions, the right side of our brain releases distress signals. When we put words to the pain we're experiencing, the left side of the brain releases calming signals to the right side of our brain, soothing its distress. When we put words to the pain we've endured, it makes those experiences less painful.

Sharing our experiences with others begins the process of healing. This must be why James told us to confess our sins to one another that we may be healed (James 5:16). I don't think this scripture only reflects our need to confess what we've done wrong, but also to confess what wrongs have been done to us. As we share our words with others, we find healing. This is why therapy is so beautifully powerful. It embodies the spiritual space God gives us to heal in a physical and tangible way.

STARTING THERAPY, DOING THE WORK

Therapy is not evidence of your mistrust in God's power; it is evidence of your trust in it. Just as God uses doctors to heal our bodies, God uses trained and licensed therapists to heal the wounds of our minds and souls. As Christians, we are called to "use whatever gift you have received to serve others, as faithful stewards of God's grace in its various forms" (1 Peter 4:10). Therapists, psychologists, and mental health professionals have been given the gift and professional training to discern the wounds of the mind and the heart and to heal them through the knowledge, wisdom, and skills God has blessed them with.

For those of us who believe in Jesus, therapy is a space where we allow Him to do the beautiful, powerful, and personal work of healing us mentally and emotionally so we can be strengthened spiritually to live out the authentic selves He purposed us to be. The discernment and personal comfort I experienced in therapy gave me reference for the comfort of the Holy Spirit when I felt far away from God. The advocacy and care I received reminded me of Jesus, when I struggled to remember He was good. The confidentiality, trust, and kindness helped me to experience safety, reminding me of what God was offering me as a Father.

In therapy we get to see and participate in the transforming work of Jesus in our lives.

GOD WON'T COME AS YOU EXPECT

How does God heal us? The answer is: in many ways.

The process of healing trauma requires that we revisit, in one way or another, the most terrifying and terrorizing moments of our lives. It requires that we give our mind, body, and spirit permission to keep growing by allowing our brain to become unstuck in the place we last processed pain—through words, through movement, through tears, through screams, through joy, through many means.

As a therapist, the modalities I primarily use for helping people resolve trauma are wholistic and somatic. My approach to trauma therapy always includes the mind, body, and soul. We didn't think ourselves into our wounds. We experienced them in a way that affected our minds and manifested in our bodies. This doesn't mean words aren't helpful in the healing process, but it does mean that sometimes we need more than words to process our pain. Jesus also healed with His physical posture. He stood next to the people others were ashamed to be seen with. Jesus touched the people deemed untouchable and laid hands on those who were seen to be unclean. In His life, Jesus' actions healed as much as His words did.

I help my clients process and heal their trauma in a way that mirrors the way they were wounded. This creates what's called a *corrective emotional experience*.

Let's say you had a friendship that was going well. But after you shared your hopes and dreams with this friend, they immediately shot them down, telling you how immature and silly they were. Such an experience is absolutely heartbreaking. To avoid that heartbreak, you may find yourself avoiding sharing your dreams with any new friends you make.

The problem is, the wound of dismissal and discouragement will never heal until you build the courage to share your dream with a friend again (maybe not the same one) and experience something different than you did with the first friend. Sharing your dream with a friend who responds with encouragement and support helps correct the emotional wounds that were created when the first friend let you down.

Does that mean that you have to go tell another friend about your dreams immediately? No! It is okay to take time to process the pain of being dismissed. Forgiveness is a gift, but trust must be earned. It's okay to incrementally build trust with people around you by sharing only what feels safe in the moment. But I believe the pinnacle of healing our wounds looks like revisiting the situations that wounded us most, going back into the room with the monsters in it, and standing "ten toes down" in territory that once broke us.

Please know that I'm not telling you to confront an abuser, or to revisit situations of assault. Everyone's process is different and intensely personal (which is why having a therapist to cater to your personal needs is important). What I am saying is that restoration will mean that you're able to do what you couldn't do before you were so deeply wounded. Your healing will look like God correcting the fractures of trust, confidence, self-esteem, creativity, spontaneity, joy, and love in your life, fractures from traumatic situations that have taken away your ability to engage.

Though there are many forms of effective therapy that you can read about in various places, some of the most powerful ways I've seen God correct deep emotional wounds are through EMDR, psychodrama, experiential forms of therapy, and other forms of somatic processing, which is simply processing information through connecting to the experiences it creates in both the mind and the body.

EMDR

EMDR (Eye Movement Desensitization and Reprocessing) therapy is a therapeutic model for those experiencing emotional distress from past traumatic experiences. Clinicians help clients decrease their distress levels related to past pain by utilizing and optimizing the body's natural mental processing system.

Have you ever noticed someone pacing back and forth or alternating hands as they twist a gum wrapper while having a hard conversation? What they're doing is called *bilateral stimulation* (which simply means stimulation of both sides of the brain). When we move one side of our body, it stimulates one side of the brain. When we use the other side of our body, it stimulates the other side of the brain. The left side of our brain processes words, logic, and language, while the right side of our brain processes emotions, meaning, attention, and other abstract things.

Have you ever logically known something was hurtful, but couldn't connect to the emotional reality of it? Your left brain was probably heavily activated. Have you ever felt deep and intense sadness but were not able to express why you felt it or what caused it? Your right brain was probably heavily activated.

EMDR rhythmically activates both sides of the brain through bilateral stimulation. Bilateral stimulation can be walking, running, or riding a bike. In therapy it's often simply tapping alternate sides of your body, hearing sounds in alternate ears, or allowing your eyes to follow the therapist's hand as it moves from left to right. Some therapists also utilize light bars that have beams of light moving from left to right, which the client follows with their eyes.

Before the bilateral stimulation, a counseling session would include much of what we did at the beginning of this book. We identify the moments that hurt deeply and then extract the negative core belief that came from it. For a client who can't clearly identify the moments that wounded them, we may identify the negative core belief first.

For every thought or belief we have, there is a neurological pathway that acts like a street in our brain. Let's call that street anxiety. For Warren, the patient and study subject we first met in chapter 4, the neurological pathways that touched on his performance in school also connected to his parents' divorce. EMDR would address all the ways his anxiety manifested, based on his neural networking.

As the client is reminded of painful moments through thoughts, images, and sensations that come up during bilateral stimulation, they experience an opportunity to process that pain with a therapist intermittently. They may even experience the presence of the Holy Spirit (like I did!) in their flashbacks, which become increasingly less painful. This process resolves the emotional pain of the past by resolving the neurological pain distress in the brain and body.

EMDR isn't hypnosis; it's a trauma-focused psychotherapy that is one of the most studied and successful treatments for PTSD (post-traumatic stress disorder) in the world. It's also utilized as one of the primary therapeutic interventions for combat veterans in the United States. It doesn't make you forget what you've been through, but it does desensitize you to the overwhelming emotions that come from unprocessed traumatic moments. It helps clients discover the lies they carried into their lives from their past trauma. It allows them to use the wisdom of the present to process the pain of the past. It also allows them to glean wisdom from the worst moments of their lives and apply it to the present, as it fuels hope for the future. EMDR is an incredibly transformative modality for trauma survivors.

I began my own process of EMDR as a client back in 2017, and I'm still processing my wounds that way today. As a clinician it's easy to write about the theoretical principles of healing—but going through it is a different matter. Going through it will make you forget everything you ever learned as a professional. After each EMDR session, the therapist "closes" with the client by helping them draw on a resource of a memory or internal image of some thing or place that makes them feel safe. Similar to what we did when we addressed our positive core belief, we use imagination to develop hope and instill safety.

I always tell my clients that "processing will continue" after our sessions, because in our short time together we brought back to the front of our attention some difficult experiences. Beyond bringing them to mind, we've activated our body's memories of those hard times. Remember when I mentioned the physical effects of trauma? Some of those symptoms can resurface. You may feel exhausted, though you've gotten a full night of sleep. You may feel deep sadness or intense rage. All these emotions now have a space to be processed, fully experienced, and cleared out from the body that has been holding on to it.

In every memory God brought up with me, His presence was clear. When my therapist would prompt me to imagine a safe person being in the room after one of my sexual assaults, I saw Jesus there in my heart and mind. Holding me as I wept. In my EMDR, my faith was renewed. I didn't just hear Bible verses; I got to experience Jesus' presence in my worst moments as I dared to look back.

Once the client has finished processing their negative core belief and the pain it brought up, they can begin to process their positive core belief. In this processing, the client recalls moments of the past that validate their positive truth and ignite their imagination, so they can begin to see a beautifully renewed life ahead of them, one that reflects the truth of who they are in Christ. This processing is the psychological reflection of Jeremiah 29:11, "'For I know the plans I have for you,' declares the LORD, 'plans to prosper you and not to harm you, plans to give you hope and a future.'"

Unfortunately, many church traditions are skeptical of EMDR simply because they don't understand it. Some call it witchcraft; some call it snake oil. But it's just harnessing a biological process, created by God Himself as He intricately and beautifully fashioned the systems of our bodies. It's a reflection of how God has already hardwired our bodies and brains for healing. Truly, we are fearfully and wonderfully made.

PSYCHODRAMA

Psychodrama is, in my opinion, one of the most powerful methods of mental and emotional healing and restoration. I believe this is because, in order to engage in it, we open our heart and mind to the creativity and trust God designed us for. It expands our understanding of God and shows that His love and redemption truly have no limits.

I shared a little about my psychodrama experience at an Onsite Workshop earlier. It changed my life. So much so that I began to train in psychodrama and now use it as the main modality of my OASIS Mental Health Intensive and Retreat. I host this retreat twice a year, and every year lives are changed. Psychodrama is the process of bringing painful and confusing emotional moments into the present through dramatization. The movement and acting that psychodrama requires activates the somatic nervous system, allowing it to heal from the effects of trauma. Each person gets to set the proverbial stage with moments of their lives that wounded them, moments they want to make sense of and resolve.

Psychodrama is usually done in groups, sometimes with strangers or friends playing the roles of the people involved in the painful memories. The subject then gets to direct each person as they replay those painful moments. But two beautiful key things happen: First, they get to stop the scene whenever they want and emotionally process what they thought, felt, or internalized in those moments, as they gain insight. Second, they get to invite whomever they want into the scene. Some people choose their grandmother, some choose a best friend, most people I work with invite Jesus. I wish I could describe to you what it's like to see someone fall into the arms of the person who plays Jesus. The physical posture brings so much light to their emotional pain. It's powerful, it's vulnerable, and the room is electric with the Holy Spirit. It brings tears to my eyes writing about it. The roles each person is called to play always draw them deeper into their own healing, as their perspectives are widened and empathy is deepened through playing a role for someone else's healing.

During my psychodrama piece, I remember staying on that floor for what felt like forever. I didn't want to let go of the feeling. I didn't want the experience to end. I was used to being comforted for small amounts of time, then urged to get up and go about my day. But each person held their post on that floor. Not a single person got up. Even when my tears stopped, even when my breathing slowed, even as my eyes took in the room around me, wide and aware, those people stayed right there as I held on to them.

I could feel the discomfort rising inside me. *They must be uncomfortable. I bet they want to get up.*

But I felt the Holy Spirit inviting me into a new pattern of letting people love me at my lowest and of staying right there. And I wanted to stay—it just felt *too* good. The longer I stayed, the more intensely I felt God's love. My heart was opened wider and wider, exposed to the truth of how vast and unimaginably unfathomable God's love for me was. Even when I wasn't in present distress, I was still getting love—a profound truth I didn't grasp until after that moment.

I thought to myself, *If absolute strangers can love me like this, how much more would the One who knows and created me?*

On that floor my ear touched the chest of Jesus, attuned to His heartbeat. As the clouds of unprocessed anger and sadness passed, I was reminded that the sun never leaves. On the clearest day and in the fiercest storm, the sun stays in the same place.

EXPERIENTIAL THERAPIES

Experiential therapies are forms of therapy that allow clients to use expressive tools, activities, and other methods to connect to, reenact, and/or re-create specific situations from past and present experiences in their lives. Experiential activities are powerful because they bring our physical, emotional, and spiritual realities into the present space we're in so we can address them all at once.

In 2018, I began to do some research on the effects of stillness, diaphragmatic breathing (belly breathing), and nonreligious meditation on the brain. I found that many of the key evidence-based benefits of these psychological activities could easily be integrated into spiritual disciplines that I'd been utilizing in my personal life. When people ask me what spiritual disciplines are, I usually say prayer is about speaking to and hearing from God, Scripture is for learning about God, and spiritual disciplines are about experiencing God.

Many of my clients had all the brain knowledge of who God was and how good He was, but they didn't know Him to be those things *to them*. I once heard that the longest distance to travel is the eighteen inches between your head and your heart. I believe that's 100 percent true.

My clients had heard so many times to take their pain to Jesus or bring it to the altar because He cares, but no one had taught them *how* to do that. Combining the centuries-old Christian practice of spiritual disciplines with evidence-based calming methods, I created a list of what I call "Christian Coping Skills." These include practices like biblically-based guided meditation, breath prayer, and centering prayer.

In combining simple evidence-based practices with ancient

Christian traditions, I found that clients got to activate the physical, emotional, and spiritual realities of their pain while simultaneously interacting with the Holy Spirit and God in a way that was completely personally driven. With these Christian Coping Skills, they got to bring their thoughts, feelings, and actions to God and, in real time, experience His grace, mercy, and compassion for their pain.

THE LIFE AHEAD OF YOU

No matter what path you take toward healing, know that there is a beautiful life ahead of you. The bad news is, you've been wounded. You have had your heart broken, abandoned, abused, forsaken, and belittled.

But the good news is, there is restoration for you. The good news is, there is nothing God can't and won't use to pave the path of abundance for you. The dreams of your heart are not God taunting you but are personal prophecies of better days to come, no matter how old you are and no matter what's happened to you. The identity that was buried under fear, shame, and unworthiness is being dug up, like a treasure in a field, one worth selling all the riches of the world for.

The story God is writing through your life is one of redemption, of healing, of intimacy, of rest, gentleness, tenderness, and abundance. God hasn't forgotten about you. God isn't ashamed of you. He doesn't laugh at how minimal and trivial your pain may seem, like people of your past may have done. He mourns with you, weeps with you, and offers you tenderness that's more relentless than the terror you've been living in.

A counselor once said something to me I'll never forget: "There has never truly been a fight between light and darkness. You've never seen someone flip on a light switch and watched light and darkness wrestle or fight. When light comes, darkness flees; it has no choice."

I would add that when light comes in, it transforms the darkness. The darkness doesn't scoot over for light, giving it room; it doesn't escape to another place—it literally transforms into the light that meets the space.

The tenderness of God is transforming and will continue to transform your darkest moments into light that will become a lamp unto your feet to light your path of healing.

Conclusion

THROUGH THE MUD

A client once told me that healing felt like being a lotus. She loved flowers and decided in one of our last sessions to tell me about this incredible flower. Lotus flowers grow in still bodies of water, like lakes and ponds. The lotus flower's roots sink deep into some of the thickest mud and some of the dirtiest, muddiest water. The lotus grows in and through the mud, reaching up to forty-nine inches toward the sun and the surface of the water, to bloom. Once it does reach the surface, it opens its petals one by one, taking its time to expose itself to the fresh air and the sun it so diligently strived for.

Every night, the lotus flower closes and retreats to the mud where it came from. And in the morning, it journeys again, through the mud, muck, and mire to find the face of the sun again—to find the cool of the morning air. And when it appears at the surface, it's spotless, holding no evidence that it spent all morning rising through the dense mud.

The lotus flower is resilient, like no other flower. Its seeds can survive droughts of more than two hundred years and can begin to grow after being dormant for thousands of years. Though they can face the harshest environments and endure the hardest trials, they remain delicate.

You, friend, are a lotus.

You are beautifully intricate—delicate, yet powerfully resilient. Whether you were born into the mud of trauma or found yourself stuck in it later in life, you don't have to live in it. You can break free of the daily patterns that hold you to the bottom of the waters, in the thick of the mud.

The tenderness of God will meet you where you are. It will give you the courage to venture through the darkness. It will fill every valley of sorrow and level every mountain of shame. It will teach you how to reach for more, to search for the sun. As you embark on the winding journey of healing and restoration called life, some days you'll be drawn to the mud of your past trauma to mourn, to grieve, to learn, to understand, and to gain wisdom for your present.

Every day you'll be called by the rising of the sun, to find the Son. To open your heart to Him as slowly as you need to, like petals opening one by one.

I pray you take the journey of healing ahead of you. The journey of tears and triumphs. A journey of shaping and molding. Of trying and failing and letting yourself be loved. Of breaking old patterns as you intentionally and delicately build new ones that align with who you really are. It's a path that will transform your everyday life as God challenges your norms, uproots your past, and plants new seeds that can't be swept away by the storms of life or plucked out by the voice of fear.

I pray that, as God opens your heart to the patterns that keep you from Him and from your authentic self, finding your way into His presence would become a new, reflexive pattern. One that aligns with who God calls you to be and the life He's called you to live.

I pray that you, like the lotus, would abide in still waters, being as delicate and tender to yourself as God has been to you. May you, every morning, grow through the mud to find the Son.

Amen.

Appendix A

GENESIS REVIEW

CHAPTER 2

Verse 15 tells us that we are called to work and that God trusts humanity to take care of creation.

Verse 16 tells us that God wants humanity to experience freedom.

Verse 17 reveals that God doesn't want humanity to die, which is why He commanded Adam not to eat certain fruit.

Verse 18 tells us God cares about our loneliness. This verse implies that we can be lonely in the presence of God if we're not also around other humans (God said, "I will make a helper suitable for him," even though Adam was surrounded by God and creation).

Verse 19: God trusts us and values our creativity. God didn't give Adam the names of the animals; rather, He told Adam to name them. How many of us, in Adam's situation, would have said, "God, just tell me what to name the animals, and I'll do it"? Sometimes beneath our appearance of commitment and obedience to God is fear and a denial of the gifts of creativity and spontaneity God designed in us.

Verse 20 again emphasizes that God designed us to enjoy human relationships. Though Adam had all these animals, none were suitable. Because they weren't like him, none could relate with or connect to him on his level. God doesn't intend for us to feel lonely.

Verse 21 tells us that God cares about our pain. God put Adam to sleep before removing his rib because He never intended for us to feel pain and doesn't delight in it when we do.

Verse 23 communicates to us that when Adam met Eve, he felt close to her. He was drawn to her because of their alikeness (as God designed).

Verse 24 tells us Adam and Eve were unified.

Verse 25 makes it clear that Adam and Eve felt no shame. God never intended for us to feel shame about ourselves, nor did He intend for us to shame others.

CHAPTER 3

Verse 7 tells us Adam and Eve noticed their nakedness and felt shame. They used fig leaves to cover themselves.

Verse 8: When they heard the Lord, they felt fear and hid among the trees. Rather than drawing near to God, they tried to escape His presence, because they were afraid.

Verses 9–10: When God asked where they were, Adam responded that he had heard God, was afraid, and hid himself.

Verses 11–12: God asked Adam and Eve who had told them they were naked, then asked if they had eaten from the forbidden tree. Rather than answering the question, Adam blamed Eve and God, saying, "The woman *you* put here with me" gave him the fruit (emphasis added).

Appendix B

EMOTION WHEEL

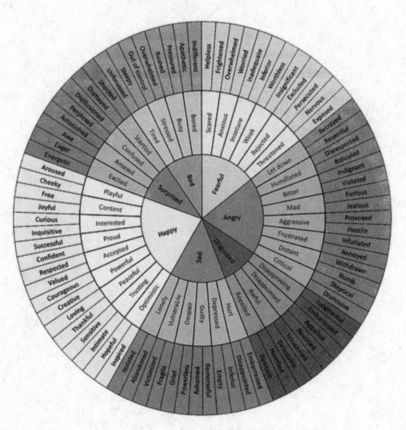

"Feelings Wheel," https://feelingswheel.com.

ACKNOWLEDGMENTS

This book is an answered prayer.

A promise that came to fruition.

Evidence that pain can become purpose.

Proof that tenderness transforms.

Thank You, God, for giving me courage to live.

Thank you to every therapist and client I've had. Your courage and wisdom shaped me. This book is ours.

Thank you, Kyle, for believing the world of me.

Thank you, Levi and Makai, for teaching me how to be free.

Thank you, Kofi, Daniel, and Odua, for being the best siblings in the world.

Thank you, Mommy and Daddy, for giving me a fighting chance in this world. For teaching me strength, determination, and perseverance. This is your legacy.

Thank you, Stephanie and Andrea, for believing in me.

NOTES

Chapter I: Trauma: How Did My Past Affect Me?

1. *Merriam-Webster*, s.v. "trauma *(n.)*," accessed November 11, 2022, https://www.merriam-webster.com/dictionary/trauma.
2. Marjie L. Roddick, "Big T and Little t Trauma and How Your Body Reacts to It," GoodTherapy, October 19, 2015, https://www.goodtherapy.org/blog/big-t-and-little-t-trauma-and-how-your-body-reacts-to-it-1019154.
3. Chun Shen et al., "Associations of Social Isolation and Loneliness with Later Dementia," *Neurology* 99, no. 2 (July 2022): e164–e175, https://doi.org/10.1212/WNL.0000000000200583.
4. Livia Tomova et al., "Acute Social Isolation Evokes Midbrain Craving Responses Similar to Hunger," *Nature Neuroscience* 23, no. 12 (December 2020): 1597–1605, https://doi.org/10.1038/s41593-020-00742-z.
5. For a verse-by-verse evaluation of this scripture, see the Genesis review in Appendix A of this book.

Chapter 2: Negative Patterns: Why Can't I Change?

1. D. O. Hebb, *The Organization of Behavior: A Neuropsychological Theory* (New York: Wiley & Sons, 1949).
2. Johan Denollet et al., "Anger, Suppressed Anger, and Risk of Adverse Events in Patients with Coronary Artery Disease," *American Journal of Cardiology* 105, no. 11 (June 2010): 1555–60, https://doi.org/10.1016/j.amjcard.2010.01.015.

3. Kalanit Grill-Spector, Richard Henson, and Alex Martin, "Repetition and the Brain: Neural Models of Stimulus-Specific Effects," *Trends in Cognitive Sciences* 10, no. 1 (January 2006): 14–23, https://doi .org/10.1016/j.tics.2005.11.006.

4. Anne Trafton, "Distinctive Brain Patterns Help Habits Form," *Neuroscience News*, February 8, 2018, https://neurosciencenews .com/habit-brain-patterns-8456/.

Chapter 3: Confronting the Past: Why Can't I Enjoy the Present?

1. Diane Langberg (@DianeLangberg), Twitter, March 1, 2022, 11:03 a.m., https://twitter.com/DianeLangberg/status/1498705484622315522.

2. "Early Childhood Trauma Re-Wires the Brain, Increasing Risk for Depression," *Newswise*, March 4, 2018, https://www.newswise.com /articles/early-childhood-trauma-re-wires-the-brain,-increasing-risk -for-depression.

3. "About the CDC-Kaiser ACE Study," Centers for Disease Control and Prevention, last reviewed April 6, 2021, https://www.cdc.gov /violenceprevention/aces/about.html.

Chapter 4: Facing Fear: Why Am I So Afraid?

1. Tian Dayton, *Trauma and Addiction: Ending the Cycle of Pain Through Emotional Literacy* (New York: Simon and Schuster, 2010), 15–17.

2. *Merriam-Webster*, s.v. "terror *(n.)*," accessed November 21, 2022, https://www.merriam-webster.com/dictionary/terror.

3. *Britannica*, s.v. "amygdala *(n.)*," accessed November 21, 2022, https://www.britannica.com/science/amygdala.

4. "Understanding the Stress Response," Harvard Health, July 6, 2020, https://www.health.harvard.edu/staying-healthy/understanding -the-stress-response.

5. "Deep Breathing and Relaxation," University of Toledo Counseling Center, accessed November 21, 2022, https://www.utoledo.edu /studentaffairs/counseling/anxietytoolbox/breathingandrelaxation. html.

6. "Integrating EMDR into Your Clinical Practice," EMDR Consulting, LLC, 61.

7. Tamaki Amano and Motomi Toichi, "The Role of Alternating Bilateral Stimulation in Establishing Positive Cognition in EMDR Therapy: A Multi-Channel Near-Infrared Spectroscopy Study," *PLoS One* 11, no. 10 (2016): e0162735, https://doi.org/10.1371%2Fjournal.pone.0162735.

Chapter 5: Investigating Identity: Why Is It So Hard to Love Myself?

1. *APA Dictionary of Psychology*, s.v. "transference *(n.)*," accessed November 21, 2022, https://dictionary.apa.org/transference.

2. Hilary Jacobs Hendel, "When a Relationship Ruptures," *Psychology Today*, July 1, 2020, https://www.psychologytoday.com/us/blog/emotion-information/202007/when-relationship-ruptures.

Chapter 6: Discovering the Truth: How Does God Respond to My Trauma?

1. "Compassion," BibleProject, September 1, 2020, YouTube video, https://www.youtube.com/watch?v=qJEtyAiAQik.

Chapter 7: Recognizing Triggers: Why Do I React This Way?

1. *APA Dictionary of Psychology*, s.v. "trigger *(n.)*," accessed November 25, 2022, https://dictionary.apa.org/trigger.

2. Michelle Yarwood, "Physiological Measures of Emotion," chap. 7 in *Psychology of Human Emotion: An Open Access Textbook* (Pennsylvania State University, last updated December 30, 2022), https://psu.pb.unizin.org/psych425/chapter/744/.

Chapter 8: Grieving the Loss: What Do I Do with the Pain?

1. Dan J. Tomasulo, "What Is Psychodrama?," *Psychology Today*, November 25, 2010, https://www.psychologytoday.com/us/blog/the-healing-crowd/201011/what-is-psychodrama.

2. *APA Dictionary of Psychology*, s.v. "grief *(n.)*," accessed November 21, 2022, https://dictionary.apa.org/grief.

3. "Chronic Stress Puts Your Health at Risk," Mayo Clinic, July 8, 2021, https://www.mayoclinic.org/healthy-lifestyle/stress -management/in-depth/stress/art-20046037.

4. Dan Diegel, "Mindsight," accessed November 21, 2022, https://drdansiegel.com/mindsight/.

5. Adele Ahlberg Calhoun, *Spiritual Disciplines Handbook: Practices That Transform Us* (Downers Grove, IL: InterVarsity Press, 2009), 204, 207.

Chapter 9: Moving Forward: How Do I Begin Healing?

1. *APA Dictionary of Psychology*, s.v. "automatic thoughts," accessed November 21, 2022, https://dictionary.apa.org/automatic-thoughts.

2. "The Number One Habit to Develop in Order to Feel More Positive," Amen Clinics, August 16, 2016, https://www.amenclinics .com/blog/number-one-habit-develop-order-feel-positive/.

3. Daniel Amen, *Change Your Brain, Change Your Life* (New York: Crown Publishing, 2015).

Chapter 10: Trusting Others with My Pain: What If I Can't Do It Alone?

1. Dan Siegel, "Name It to Tame It," Dalai Lama Center for Peace and Education, December 8, 2014, YouTube video, https://www .youtube.com/watch?v=ZcDLzppD4Jc.

ABOUT THE AUTHOR

Kobe Campbell is a Charlotte-based, Ghanaian American licensed clinical mental health counselor (LCMHC), trauma specialist, writer, and speaker. Named one of Charlotte's Most Influential Women by *Charlotte Lately Magazine* and awarded Rising Star Under 30 by *WILMA* magazine, Kobe is a decorated and highly sought-after speaker, facilitator, and educator.

Kobe is founder of The Healing Circle Therapy & Wellness Center in Charlotte, North Carolina, and hosts *The Healing Circle* podcast. With a kind, compassionate, and energetic spirit, Kobe helps people discover who they are apart from what they've experienced, through therapy, support groups, speaking, retreats, organizational trainings, and more.

When Kobe isn't teaching and training, she's spending time with her husband and kids, playing her guitar, writing poetry, or traveling. She looks forward to sharing her expertise with anyone willing to learn and grow.

From the Publisher

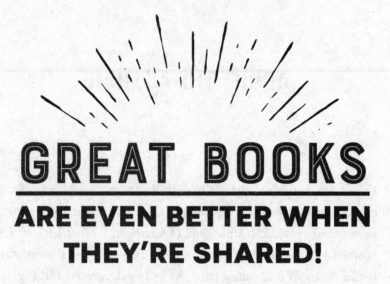

GREAT BOOKS

ARE EVEN BETTER WHEN THEY'RE SHARED!

Help other readers find this one:

- Post a review at your favorite online bookseller

- Post a picture on a social media account and share why you enjoyed it

- Send a note to a friend who would also love it—or better yet, give them a copy

Thanks for reading!